A Practical Guide to Brain Health

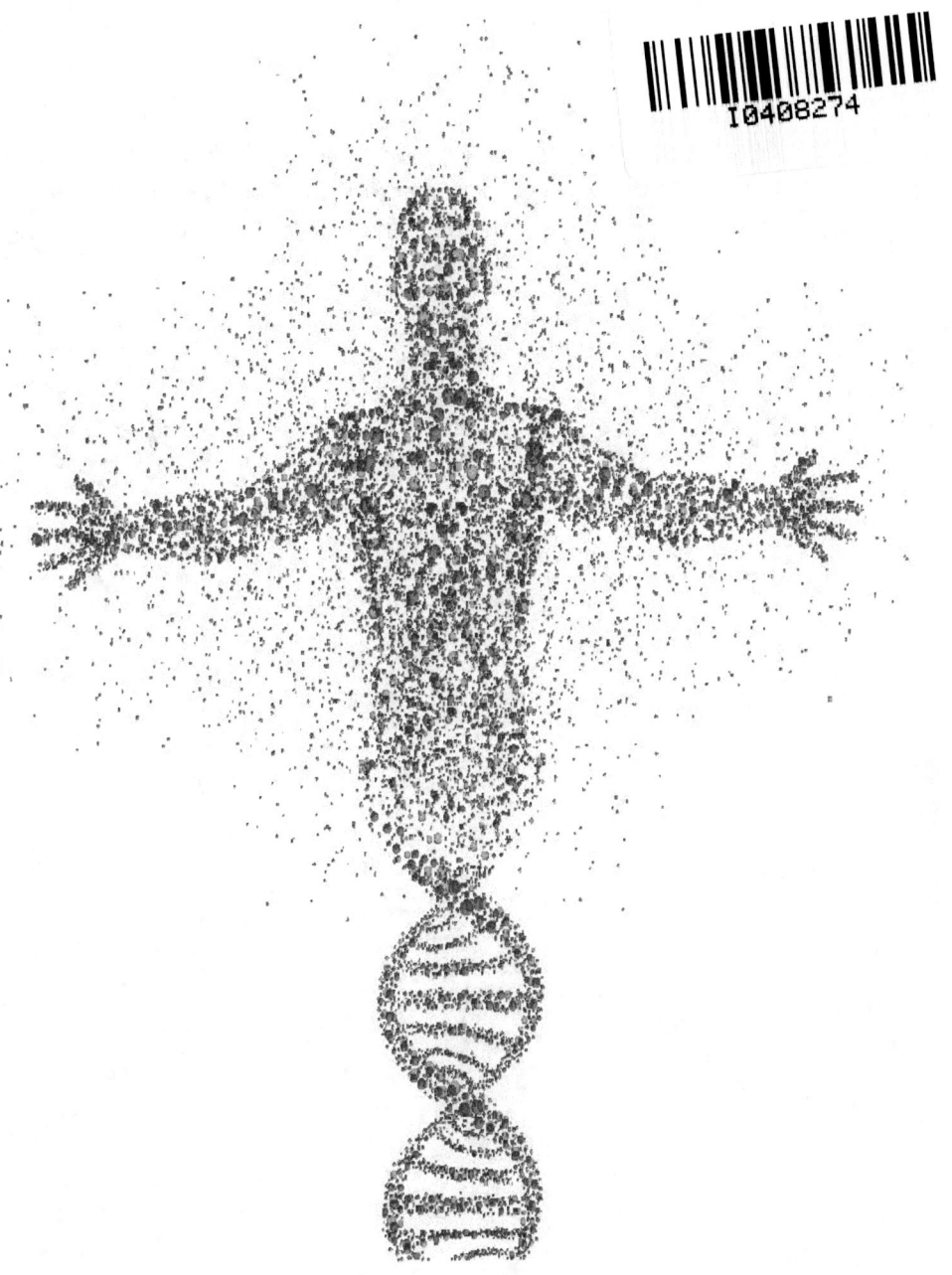

Enhancing the Growth of New Brain Cells

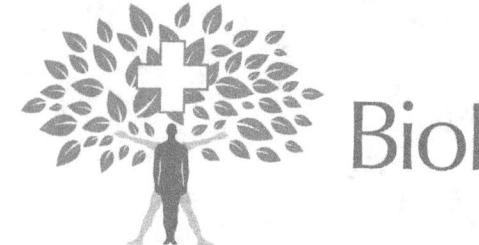

Disclaimer

The information in this book is not intended to replace a one-on-one relationship with a qualified health care professional and is not intended as medical advice. It is intended as a sharing of knowledge and information from the research and experience of the author. The author encourages you to make your own health care decisions based upon your research and in partnership with a qualified health care professional.

The author strongly recommends that any person who purchases or reads this book understand the following:

1.   The supplement (nootropics, nutraceuticals, foods, herbs and spices) approach outlined in this book is intended for adults only.   Persons under the age of 18 should not take any supplements for any reason without first consulting with a qualified health care advisor.

2.   The author shall not be held responsible in anyway for the misuse of the information contained within this book.

3.   The author strongly recommends that all persons contact his/her health care advisor before starting the suggestions outlined in this book in order to get a health care advisor's approval prior to taking any supplements (nootropics, nutraceuticals, foods, herbs and spices) discussed in this book.

4.   The author insists that if the reader has any known or suspected medical conditions, that may include but is not limited to; pregnancy, heart disease, high blood pressure, mental disorder, kidney disorder, liver disorder, immune system disorder, history of stroke, history of seizure, etc, then the reader will contact a qualified health care professional and get a qualified health care professional's approval prior to taking any of the supplements (nootropics, nutraceuticals, foods, herbs and spices) discussed in this book.

5.   The reader assumes all liability if he/she passes this information to others without fully divulging the risks and recommendations set forth in this text.

The statements in this book have not been evaluated by the Food and Drug Administration. The supplements (nootropics, nutraceuticals, foods, herbs and spices) and suggested products are not intended to diagnose, treat, cure or prevent any disease. If you are pregnant, nursing, taking medication, or have a medical condition, consult your health care professional before using the supplements (nootropics, nutraceuticals, foods, herbs and spices) and suggested products.

Table of Contents

Introduction

In 1998, neuroscientists undertook to investigate whether neurogenesis occurs in the adult human brain. They concluded that the human hippocampus retains its ability to generate neurons throughout life. Their results were published in the medical journal <u>Nature Medicine</u>.

While conducting their research, they discovered that the brain contains neural stem cells and progenitor cells which differentiate into brain neurons.

Since DNA ultimately controls the process of neurogenesis, there are specific genes that code for the production of various proteins called neurotrophins. These neurotrophins play a key role in the birth of new brain cells.

The birth of new neurons (neurogenesis) is highly related to neuroplasticity. Neuroplasticity is the ability of a particular part or region of a neuron to change in strength over time. It refers to changes in neural pathways and synapses due to changes in behavior, environment, neural processes, thinking, emotions, as well as changes resulting from bodily injury. Neuroplasticity has replaced the formerly-held position that the brain is a physiologically static organ, and explores how - and in which ways - the brain changes throughout life.

Brain atrophy is a condition in which the brain is in the process of shrinking (or a limited portion of the brain is shrinking) and that little if no neurogenesis is taking place.

If you were to look at neurogenesis as a full spectrum, you would find enhanced and optimal neurogenesis and brain atrophy as polar opposites on this spectrum.

The full spectrum would reveal that in a healthy fully optimized brain there would be enhanced neurogenesis; yet in a compromised brain there would first be neuroinflammation, then at the opposite end, brain atrophy.

This book will examine the natural substances that can be consumed in the form of Nootropics, Nutraceuticals, Foods, Herbs and Spices to maximize the state of enhanced neurogenesis and to enhance the three (3) main neurotrophins that facilitate neurogenesis. In addition, the subject of Brain Atrophy will be examined and the recommended substances that can be consumed to prevent and inhibit brain atrophy.

The intent of this book is to be a practical guide to enhancing neurogenesis for optimal brain health.

Creating New Brain Cells: Neurogenesis

The birth of new brain cells (neurogenesis) continues throughout life in the brain, in particular the dentate gyrus region of the hippocampus.

The hippocampus produces roughly 700 new brain cells each day.   This corresponds to an annual turnover of 1.75% of the neurons within the renewing fraction, with a modest decline during aging.

Neurogenesis is generated in two regions of the adult brain:

The subventricular zone (SVZ) lining the lateral ventricles (Figure 1.1)

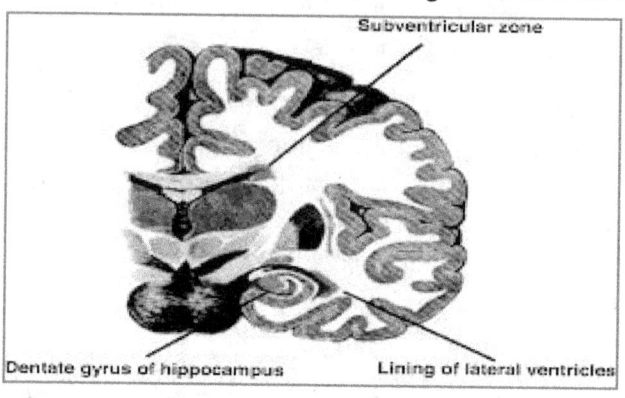

Figure 1.1 Subventricular zone

The subgranular zone (SGZ), part of the dentate gyrus of hippocampus. (Figure 1.2)

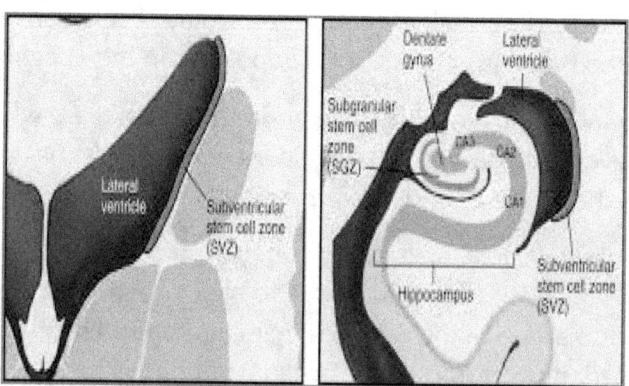

Figure 1.2   Subgranular zone

There are some neuroscientists that claim that adult neurogenesis may also occur in the neocortex.

Neurogenesis can have tremendous functional significance to the healthy adult brain. In the aging adult, hippocampal function declines with potential memory dysfunction. This may due to the fact that neurogenesis is substantially reduced in the hippocampus in the aging adult.

If neurogenesis in the hippocampus continues throughout life, then one would presume that the size of hippocampus would increase in size. However, this is not the case since the rate of neuron death balances out the proliferation.

The hippocampus does experience cerebral atrophy in the aging adult, wherein the hippocampus shrinks in size. If neurogenesis is not enhanced new neurons proliferate, then the hippocampus may experience shrinkage. Some MRI studies have reported shrinkage of the hippocampus in elderly people, but other studies have failed to reproduce this finding.

Neurogenesis is also linked to changes in neuroplasticity, which is referring to changes in synapses and neural pathways in the brain.

What is the Significance of Adult Neurogenesis

Adult neurogenesis plays significant roles in synaptic plasticity, memory, and mood regulation.

Decreased neurogenesis in the hippocampus via aging or stress has been implicated in the pathogenesis of cognitive deficits, anxiety and depression. Neurogenesis not only plays an important role in antidepressant action but also plays a role in ameliorating various pathological disease conditions.

Table 1.1 Functional Significance of Adult Neurogenesis

Significance of Neurogenesis		
Function	**Significance**	**Notes/Reference(s)**
Synaptic Plasticity		
	Neurogenesis shares some particular functional, information processing roles that benefit from neurogenetic plasticity in addition to the universal system of synaptic plasticity	
Memory		
	Hippocampal adult neurogenesis is important for memory	
Learning		
	Hippocampal adult neurogenesis is important for learning	
Alzheimer's disease		
	Decreased hippocampal neurogenesis can lead to development of Alzheimer's disease	
Depression		
	Decreased neurogenesis is	

	associated with the onset of depression	
Stress		
	Suppression of adult neurogenesis can lead to an increased HPA-axis stress response in mildly stressful situations.	

Conditions and Substances that decrease the proliferation of neurogenesis

Other than normal aging, there are certain conditions and substances that act to inhibit and decrease the proliferation of neurogenesis.

Table 1.2 Decreased and Inhibited Proliferation of Neurogenesis

Decreased and Inhibited Proliferation of Neurogenesis		
Substance/Condition	**Effect**	**Notes/Reference(s)**
Caffeine		
	Physiologically relevant doses of caffeine can significantly depress adult hippocampal neurogenesis	
Ethanol (Alcohol)		
	Chronic alcohol exposure reduces hippocampal neurogenesis and dendritic growth of newborn neurons	
High fat diet		
	Data indicates that high dietary fat (corn oil) intake can disrupt hippocampal neurogenesis, probably through an increase in serum corticosterone levels	
Homocysyteine		
	Increased homocysteine inhibits proliferation of neuronal precursors in the mouse adult brain by impairing the basic fibroblast growth factor signaling cascade	
Sucrose		
	Excessive consumption of sucrose may lower the production of Brain Derived Neurotrophic Factor (BDNF)	
High fructose		

	Fructose solution administered for four weeks and observed a 40% reduction in BrdU/NeuN-immunoreactive cells in the hippocampal dentate gyrus.	
Chronic Stress		
	Chronic stress can result in a decreased neuronal proliferation.	
Depression		
	Depression can result in a decreased neuronal proliferation	
Lack of Sleep		
	There is a link between lack of sleep and a reduction in rodent hippocampal neurogenesis	
Microbiome		
	Microbes in the gut also influence hippocampal levels of BDNF.	

The Nootropics, Nutraceuticals, Foods and Herbs that enhance neurogenesis

What influences neurogenesis and what can we do to enhance the natural process of neurogenesis?

There are two direct actions that can be taken to enhance neurogenesis.

The first is biochemical intervention through certain and selected nootropics, nutraceuticals, foods, herbs and spices. (**See Table 1.3**)

The second is through certain behavioral activities. (**See Table 1.4**)

Table 1.3 Nootropics/Nutraceuticals/Foods/Herbs/Spices that Enhance Neurogenesis

Neurogenesis		
Category	**Nootropics/Nutraceuticals/ Foods/Herbs**	**Notes/Reference(s)**
Amino Acids		
	Taurine	
	Proline-rich polypeptide	
Foods		
	Grape Seed Extract	
	Blueberries	
Herbs		
	Ahwagandha	
	Green Tea	
	Gastrodia elata (Gastrodin)	
	Cannabinoids	
Hormones		
	Testosterone	
	Pregnenolone	
	Melatonin	
Krebs Cycle Chemical		

	Oxaloacetate		
Lipids			
	Omega 3 Fatty Acids		
	Docosahexaenoic acid (DHA)		
	Queen Bee Acid		
Minerals			
	Zinc		
	Lithium Orotate		
Nootropics			
	Galantamine		
Nucleic Compound			
	Uridine-5'-monophosphate		
Polyphenols			
	Curcumin		
	Apigenin		
Quinones			
	Pyrroloquinoline quinone (PQQ))		
Spices			
	Turmeric (Curcuma longa)	aromatic-turmerone (aka ar-turmerone)	
	Sage (Apigenin content)		
Vitamins			
	Thiamine		
	Folic Acid		
	Vitamin A		

The behavioral actions that can be taken to enhance neurogenesis

Neuroscience recognizes certain behavioral actions that can be taken to enhance neurogenesis.

Table 1.4 Behavioral Actions to Enhance Neurogenesis

Behavior	Effect	Notes/Reference(s)
Aerobic exercise		
	Physical activity in the form of voluntary exercise results in an increase in the number of newborn neurons in the hippocampus	
Meditation		
	Meditation may increase BDNF levels	
Cranial Electrical Stimulation (CES)		
	CES therapy stimulates neurogenesis by helping the brain replenish damaged brain cells with new brain cells.	
Enriched environment		
	Attaining and engaging in higher levels of thought and education, environments in which people participate in more challenging cognitively stimulating activities, results in greater cognitive reserve	Verbal/Linguistic Logical Visual/Spatial Musical/Rhythmic Bodily/Kinesthetic Nature Interpersonal Intrapersonal
Sunlight exposure		
	Increasing amounts of BDNF	

	found in the blood during months with the most sunshine	
Calorie restriction		
	Results suggest that restricted calorie intake may increase the number of divisions that neural stem and progenitor cells undergo in the aging brain	
Ketogenic diet		
	Results suggest that the KD enhances neurogenesis, which may be related to its beneficial effects on epilepsy.	
Sexual experience		
	Sexual experience promotes adult neurogenesis in the hippocampus	
Proper sleep patterns		
	Strong evidence that disruptions of sleep exceeding 24 h, by total deprivation, selective REM sleep deprivation, and chronic restriction or fragmentation, significantly inhibit cell proliferation and in some cases neurogenesis	
Learning		
	New brain cells are more likely to respond to incoming information through continual learning.	

Neurotrophins (Neurotrophic Factors)

Neurotrophins (also called Neurotrophic Factors) are a family of proteins that induce the survival, development, and function of neurons. Neurotrophic factors are secreted by target tissue and act by preventing the associated neuron from initiating programmed cell death - thus allowing the neurons to survive.

They are chemicals that assist in the stimulation and control of neurogenesis.

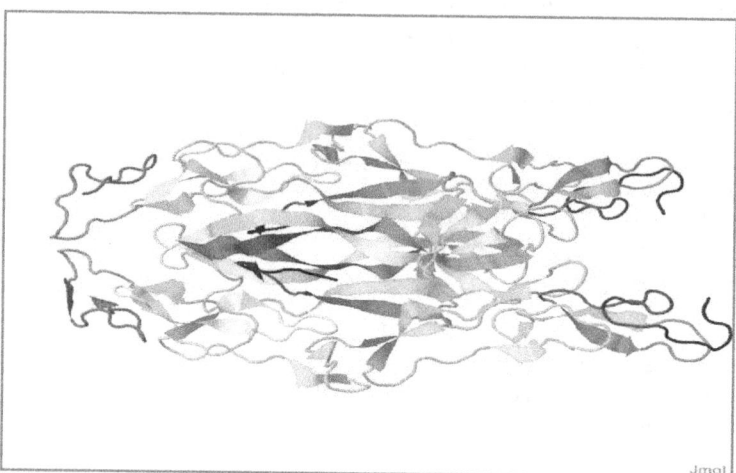

Figure 3.1   Monomer Front View of Neurotrophin

Neurotrophins consists of six structurally related neurotrophic factors:

Nerve growth factor (NGF)

Brain-derived neurotrophic factor (BDNF)

Glial Cell Line-Derived Neurotrophic Facotr (GDNF)

Ciliary neurotrophic factor (CNTF)

Neurotrophin-3 (NT-3)

Neurotrophin-4 (NT-4)

In this book, I will focus primaily on the first three (and main) neurotrophic factors, nerve growth factor (NGF), brain-derived neurotrophic factor (BDNF) and glial cell line-derived neurotrophic factor (GDNF).

Nerve Growth Factor Receptors

Nerve growth factor receptors are a group of growth factor receptors which specifically bind to neurotrophins.

There are two classes of receptors, p75 and the "Trk" family of Tyrosine kinases receptors.

It is important to maintain the proper function of nerve growth factor receptors and can be obtained with the substances in Table 2.1.

Table 2.1 Nootropics/Nutraceuticals/Foods/Herbs/Spices that Enhance the Function of NGF Receptors

NGF Receptors		
Category	**Nootropics/Nutraceuticals /Foods/Herbs/Spices**	**Notes/Reference(s)**
Amino Acids		
	Acetyl-L-Carnitine (ALCAR)	
Hormones		
	Testosterone	
	Irisin	Fibronectin type III domain-containing protein 5 also known as irisin
Vitamins		
	Alpha-GPC	

Nerve Growth Factor (NGF)

Nerve growth factor (NGF), is a protein secreted by a neuron's target cell and is critical for the survival and maintenance of sympathetic and sensory neurons.

The Nobel Prize in physiology was awarded to Stanley Cohen and Rita Levi-Montalcini in 1986 for the discovery of NGF.

Table 2.2 Biological Functions of Nerve Growth Factor (NGF)

Functions of NGF		
Function	**Effect**	**Notes/Reference(s)**
Stimulates outgrowth of axons		
	Both NGF and brain-derived neurotrophic factor (BDNF) were found to stimulate the regeneration of axons from adult DRG neurons.	
Improve memory in Alzheimer's		
	May improve memory in Alzheimer's disease	
Learning		
	Essential for learning to occur	
Compassion and Empathy		
	Significant positive correlation between levels of NGF and the intensity of compassion and empathy	
Cholinergic neurons		
	NGF stimulates the growth of cholinergic neurons	
New neurons and dendrites		
	Stimulates the synthesis of	

	endogenous proteins that lead to the growth of new neurons including their dendrites	

Table 2.3 Nootropics/Nutraceuticals/Foods/Herbs/Spices that Enhance the Function of Nerve Growth Factor (NGF)

Nerve Growth Factor		
Category	**Nootropics/Nutraceuticals /Foods/Herbs/Spices**	**Notes/Reference(s)**
Alkaloids		
	Huperzine A	
	Berberine	
Amino Acids		
	Acetyl-L-Carnitine (ALCAR)	
Fungi		
	Lions Mane	Hericium erinaceus
Herbs		
	Astragulus	
	Gotu Kola	
	Codonopsis pilosula	
	Cistanche	Cistanches Herba extract
	Ginko Biloba	
	Polygala tenuifolia	increases NGF secretion in astrocytes
	Rosemary (Carnosic Acid)	
	Ashitaba	(Angelica keiskei)
	American ginseng (Panax quinquefolius)	
	Rehmannia	

	Palmitine	
	Sesamin	
Hormones		
	Estradiol	
	Testosterone	
	Pregnenolone	
	Melatonin	
Lipids		
	(Docosahexaenoic acid (DHA)	
	Phosphatidylserine	
Nootropics		
	Noopept	
	Deprenyl	
	Hydergine	
	Idebenone	
	Nicergoline	
Nucleic Compounds		
	Uridine-5'-monophosphate	
	Triacetyluridine (TAU)	
Polyphenols		
	Quercetin	
Proteins		
	Lactoferrin	
Quinones		
	Pyrroloquinolone Quinone (PQQ)	
Spices		
	Tumeric	

Vitamins		
	Vitamin A	
	Vitamin D	

Brain-Derived Neurotrophic Factor (BDNF)

Brain-derived neurotrophic factor (BDNF) is a neurotrophic factor found originally in the brain, (it is active in the hippocampus, cortex, cerebellum, and basal forebrain) but also found in the periphery.

Brain-Derived Neurotrophic Factor (BDNF) plays a major role in neurogenesis. It also protects existing neurons and promotes the survivability of existing neurons, and encourages the growth and differentiation of new neurons and synapses through axonal and dendritic sprouting..

BDNF encourages synaptic formation which connects one neuron to another for communication between neurons which is vital for learning, thinking, memory and higher levels of brain function.

BDNF is one of the most active substances to stimulate neurogenesis.

Table 2.4 Biological Functions of Brain-Derived Neurotrophic Factor (BDNF)

Functions of BDNF		
Function	**Effect**	**Notes/Reference(s)**
Anxiety		
	BDNF may reduce Anxiety	
Panic disorder		
	Panic disorder may be evidence of reduced BDNF levels	
Appetite		
	Elevated BDNF levels may reduce appetite	
Glucose utilization		
	BDNF improves the utilization of glucose in the brain	
Depression		
	BDNF is involved in depression, such that the expression of BDNF is decreased in depressed patients.	
Memory		

	BDNF is not only necessary, but sufficient to induce a late post-acquisition phase in the hippocampus essential for persistence of long -term memory storage.	
Learning ability		
	BDNF influences higher cognitive functions and complex behaviors	
Spatial memory		
	BDNF enhances spatial memory	
Growth or neurons		
	BDNF is involved in the survival and growth of Neurons including: - Cholinergic neurons - GABAergic Neurons - Dopaminergic Neurons	
Parkinson's		
	Lower BDNF levels in early stages of the disease may be associated with pathogenic mechanisms of PD	
Schizophrenia		
	BDNF levels were significantly lower in first-episode patients with schizophrenia than in healthy control subjects	
Motor neurons		
	BDNF is involved in the survival and growth of motor nerves	

Table 2.5 Nootropics/Nutraceuticals/Foods/Herbs/Spices that Enhance the Function of BDNF

Brain-Derived Neurotrophic Factor		
Category	**Nootropics/Nutraceuticals/Foods/Herbs**	**Notes/Reference(s)**
Alkaloids		
	Huperzine A	
Amino Acids		
	L-Theanine	
	Beta-Alanine	
Food		
	Euphoria Longan (fruit/berry)	
	Blueberries	
	Cacao	
Herbs		
	Gotu Kola	
	Green Tea	
	Korean Ginseng	
	Rehmannia	
	Gynostemma pentaphyllum (Jiaogulan)	
	Gastrodia elata (Gastrodin)	
	Gedunin (Neem derivative)	
Hormones		
	Melatonin	
	Estradiol	
	Progesterone	
Lipids		

	(Docosahexaenoic acid (DHA))	
	Omega 3 Fatty Acids	
	Queen Bee Acid (Royal Jelly) (10-hydroxy-2-decenoic acid)	
Minerals		
	Magnesiun-l-threonate	
	Lithium (Lithium Orotate)	
	Zinc	
Nootropics		
	Semax	
	Noopept	
	Deprenyl	
	Hydergine	
	Nicergoline	
Polyphenols		
	7,8-dihydroxyflavone (7,8-DHF)	flavonoid
	4'-Dimethylamino-7,8-dihydroxyflavone	
	Curcumin	
	Quercetin	
Spices		
	Ceylon Cinnamon	
Vitamins		
	Vitamin A	
	Vitamin B5 (Pantethine form)	

Glial Cell Line-Derived Neurotrophic Factor (GDNF)

The GDNF family of ligands consist of four proteins:

      gial cell line-derived neurotrophic factor (GDNF)

      neurturin (NRTN)

      artemin (ARTN)

      persephin (PSPN)

Table 2.6 Biological Functions of Glial Cell Line-Derived Neurotrophic Factor (GDNF)

Functions of GDNF		
Function	**Effect**	**Notes/Reference(s)**
Dopaminergic neurons		
	GDNF promotes the survival of dopaminergic neurons in the substantia nigra of the brain	
Regenerating Axons		
	GDNF is a promising potential therapy for regenerating damaged nerves	
Neurite outgrowth		
	GDNF promotes neurite outgrowth	
Parkinson's		
	GDNF is a promising potential therapy for Parkinson's disease (due to its ability to prolong the survival of dopaminergic neurons in the substantia nigra of the brain) GDNF therapy for human Parkinson's Disease patients is presently undergoing Phase 1 clinical trials.	

Table 2.7 Nootropics/Nutraceuticals/Foods/Herbs/Spices that Enhance the Function of Glial Cell Line-Derived Neurotrophic Factor (GDNF)

Glial Cell Line DNF (GDNF)		
Category	**Nootropics/Nutraceuticals/Foods/Herbs**	**Notes/Reference(s)**
Herbs		
	Ginko Biloba	
	Rehmannia	
	Withania somnifera (Ashwagandha)	
Hormones		
	Melatonin	
Lipids		
	Royal Jelly	
Nootropics		
	Deprenyl	
Vitamins		
	Vitamin D	

Summary of Substances for Neurotrophic Factors and Neurogenesis

Table 2.8 is a summary and consolidation of the substances that can be consumed for both neurogenesis (**Table 1.3 NEURO**) and all three main neurotrophic factors (**Tables 2.3 (NGF), 2.5 (BDNF) and 2.7 GCLDN)**).

Those substances that cover more than two (2) substances are highlighted.

Table 2.8   Summary of Neurotrophic Factors and Neurogenesis

Neurotrophic Factors and Neurogenesis						
Category	Nootropics/Nutraceuticals /Foods/Herbs/Spices	NGF	BDNF	GCLDN	NEURO	Totals
Alkaloids						
	Berberine	X				1
	Huperzine A	X	X			2
Amino Acids						
	Acetyl-L-Carnitine (ALCAR)	X				1
	L-Theanine		X			1
	Beta-Alanine		X			1
	Taurine				X	1
	Proline-rich polypeptides				X	1
Food						
	Blueberries		X		X	2
	Euphoria longan		X			1
	Cacao		X			1
	Grape Seed Extract				X	1
Fungi						
	Lions Mane	X				1
Herbs						
	Astragulus	X				1

	Gotu Kola	X	X			2
	American Ginseng	X				1
	Ashwagandha			X	X	2
	Cistanche	X				1
	Codonopsis pilosula	X				1
	Ginko Biloba	X		X		2
	Gynostemma pentaphyllum (Jiaogulan)		X			1
	Gastrodia elata (Gastrodin)		X		X	2
	Polygala tenuifolia	X				1
	Rosemary	X				1
	Rehmannia	X	X	X		3
	Green Tea		X		X	2
	Korean Ginseng		X			1
	Ashitaba (Angelica keiskei)	X				1
	Palmitine	X				1
	Cannabinoids				X	1
Hormones						
	Estradiol	X	X			2
	Progesterone		X			1
	Melatonin	X	X	X	X	4
	Testosterone	X			X	2
	Pregnenolone	X			X	2
Krebs Cycle						
	Oxaloacetate				X	1
Lipids						
	Docosahexaenoic acid (DHA)	X	X		X	3
	Phosphatidylserine	X				1

	Omega 3 Fatty Acids		X		X	2
	Royal Jelly			X		1
	Queen Bee Acid (Royal Jelly) (10-hydroxy-2-decenoic acid)		X		X	2
Minerals						
	Magnesium-l-threonate		X			1
	Lithium Orotate		X		X	2
	Zinc		X		X	2
Nootropics						
	Noopept	X	X			2
	Semax		X			1
	Deprenyl	X	X	X		3
	Hydergine	X	X			2
	Nicergoline	X	X			2
	Idebenone	X				1
	Galantamine				X	1
Nucleic Compunds						
	Uridine-5'-monophosphate	X			X	2
	Triacetyluridine (TAU)	X				1
Polyphenols						
	Curcumin		X		X	2
	Quercetin	X	X			2
	7,8-dihydroxyflavone (7,8-DHF)		X			1
Proteins						
	Lactoferrin	X				1
Quinones						
	Pyrroloquinoline Quinone	X			X	2

Spices						
	Ceylon Cinnamon		X			1
	Tumeric	X				1
Vitamins						
	Vitamin A	X	X		X	3
	Vitamin B5 (Pantethine)		X			1
	Vitamin D	X		X		2
	Folic Acid				X	1
	Thiamine (Vitamin B1)				X	1
Totals		**34**	**32**	**7**	**24**	**97**

Brain Atrophy (Brain Shrinkage)

Brain atrophy, or brain shrinkage, is the opposite of neurogenesis. Brain atrophy describes a loss of neurons and the connections between them.

Brain atrophy can be categorized as either general or focal. With general brain atrophy, all of the brain shrinks. With focal brain atrophy, shrinkage of the brain affects a limited area of the brain which often results in decreased functions in the area that area controls. For example, if the cerebrum atrophizes, then conscious thought and voluntary processes may be impaired.

Even if you do not have a chronic disease, you may be losing as much as 0.4% of your brain mass every year. The rate of brain shrinkage increases with age and is a major factor in early cognitive decline and premature death. Age related cognitive decline occurs in tandem with the physical degradation of brain structure.

By the age of 60, approximately .5 to 1% of brain volume is lost per year. By the time you reach age 75, your brain is on average of 15% smaller than it was when you were in your mid-20's.

Even though brain shrinkage is progressive, a growing number of neuroscientists believe that brain shrinkage can be slowed or even reversed.

Common Causes of Brain Atrophy

Medical science has recognized a number of conditions and behaviors that cause brain atrophy.

Table 3.1 Common Causes of Brain Atrophy

Brain Atrophy		
Anatomy/Condition	**Effect**	**Notes**
Homocysteine		
	Homocysteine is a risk factor for brain atrophy. Supplementation with B vitamins that lower levels of plasma total homocysteine can slow the rate of brain atrophy in subjects with mild cognitive impairment.	
Sleep		
	Poor sleep quality was associated with reduced volume within the right superior frontal cortex in cross-sectional analyses, and an increased rate of atrophy within widespread frontal, temporal, and parietal regions in longitudinal analyses.	
Hypertension		
	Studies have shown that both high and low blood pressure (BP) may play a role in the etiology of brain atrophy. High BP in midlife has been associated with more brain atrophy later in life.	
Hypoperfusion		
	Normal aging is associated with diminished blood flow to the brain. This pathology is known as hypoperfusion and causes cell injury and death. The combination of	

	hypertension and hypoperfusion is associated with smaller brain volume.	
Type 2 Diabetes		
	New research has shown that cognitive decline in people with type 2 diabetes is likely due to brain atrophy, or shrinkage, that resembles patterns seen in the early stages of Alzheimer's disease.	
Obesity		
	Higher body mass index (BMI, a measure of obesity) is associated with lower brain volume in obese and overweight people.	
Smoking		
	Any lifetime history of smoking (even if you currently do not smoke) is associated with faster brain shrinkage in multiple brain regions, compared with people who never smoked.	
Alcohol		
	Heavy drinkers are 80% more likely than nondrinkers to sustain frontal lobe shrinkage, compared with nondrinkers,49 and 32% more likely to have enlargement of the ventricles, indicating shrinkage from within.	

The Nootropics, Nutraceuticals, Foods and Herbs that Inhibit and Prevent Brain Atrophy

Table 3.2 lists the substances that have been studied for their ability to inhibit or prevent brain atrophy.

Table 3.2 Nootropics/Nutraceuticals/Foods/Herbs/Spices that Inhibit and Prevent Brain Atrophy

Brain Atrophy		
Category	Nootropics/Nutraceuticals/Foods/Herbs/Spices	Notes/Reference(s)
Foods		
	Pomegranate	
Lipids		
	Docosahexaenoic acid (DHA)	
Polyphenols		
	Resveratrol	
Vitamins		
	B Complex Vitamins (reduces homocysteine levels)	
	Vitamin B12	

Appendix A: Definition of Certain Substances

Alkaloids

<u>Berberine</u>

Berberine from the protoberberine group of isoquinoline alkaloids.   It is found in a number of plants (roots and stems), primarily in Oregon Grape (Mahonia aquifolium) and Goldenseal (Hydrastis canadensis).   It is also found in Tinospora cordifolia stem (Guduchi).

Berberine seems to act as an herbal antidepressant and a neuroprotector against neurodegenerative disorders.

Berberine can be purchased as a standalone supplement or can be obtained through the injestion of the Oregon Grape or Goldenseal herbs.

<u>Huperzine A</u>

Huperzine A occurs as a sesquiterpene alkaloid compound found in the firmoss Huperzia serrata.

It is a potent reversible acetylcholinesterase inhibitor and has been effective in helping Alzheimer patients.   Huperzine A is very neuroprotective against glutamate and beta-amyloid pigmentation.

Amino acids

Beta-Alanine

Beta-alanine is a modified version of the amino acid alanine.

β-Alanine is the rate-limiting precursor of carnosine. Supplementation with β-alanine has been shown to increase the concentration of carnosine in muscles.

Acetyl-L-Carnitine (ALCAR)

Acetyl-L-carnitine or ALCAR, is an acetylated form of L-carnitine. The acetylated form is considered to be the most effective since it offers a higher absorption rate and bioavailability.

Taurine

Taurine is an organic acid and accounts for up to 0.1% of total human body weight.

Taurine has many fundamental biological roles, such as conjugation of bile acids, antioxidation, osmoregulation, membrane stabilization, and modulation of calcium signaling. It is essential for cardiovascular function, and development and function of skeletal muscle, the retina, and the central nervous system.

Proline-rich polypeptide

Proline-rich polypeptides are a naturally occurring mixture derived from bovine colostrum.

Proline-rich polypeptides have shown possible efficacy against various illnesses including neurodegenerative diseases such as Alzheimer's.

L-Theanine

L-Theanine is an amino acid that is typically extracted from green tea . It is similar in structure and has many of the same effects as Glutamate, a neurotransmitter in the brain that is involved in learning and memory.

L-Theanine has also been shown to promote significant cognitive improvement in alertness, arousal, and attention.

Foods

Grape Seed Extract

Grape Seed Extract contains proanthocyanidin, a bioflavanoid complex and antioxidant extracted from the seeds of common wine grape (Vitis vinifera).

It is standardized to contain at least 95% proanthocyanidins.

It is also known to contain concentrations of vitamin E, flavonoids and linoleic acid.

Euphoria Longan

Dimocarpus longan, commonly known as the longan is a tropical tree that produces edible fruit.

Euphoria Longan is a synonym of Dimocarpus longan.

Euphoria longan fruit is prescribed as a tonic and for the treatment of forgetfulness, insomnia, or palpitations caused by fright in traditional Chinese medicine.

Aqueous extract of Euphoria longan fruit enhances learning and memory, and that its beneficial effects are mediated, in part, by BDNF expression and immature neuronal survival.

Fungi

<u>Lions Mane</u>

Hericium erinaceus (also called Lion's Mane Mushroom) is an edible mushroom and medicinal mushroom in the tooth fungus group.

In traditional Chinese medicine this mushroom has long been considered a medicinal mushroom for possible anti-dementia compounds and other neuroprotective potential, including stimulating nerve cells, improved cognitive ability, stimulation of nerve growth factor, stimulated myelination and regenerated peripheral nerves.

Herbs

American Ginseng

American ginseng (Panax quinquefolius) is a herbaceous perennial plant in the ivy family.

American ginseng contains dammarane-type ginsenosides, or saponins, as the major biologically active constituents. Dammarane-type ginsenosides include two classifications: 20(S)-protopanaxadiol (PPD) and 20(S)-protopanaxatriol (PPT). American ginseng contains high levels of Rb1, Rd (PPD classification), and Re (PPT classification) ginsenosides.

Ashwagandha (Withania somnifera)

Ashwagandha is a medicinal herb in Ayurveda and includes other common names as the King of Ayurveda, Indian Ginseng, and Wintercherry.

The main chemical constituents are alkaloids and steroidal lactones. These include tropine and cuscohygrine. The leaves contain the steroidal lactones, withanolides, notably withaferin A.

Ashitaba (Angelica keiskei)

Angelica keiskei, commonly known under the Japanese name of Ashitaba (アシタバ or 明日葉, literally "Tomorrow's Leaf"), is a not frost tender perennial plant from the angelica genus.

Ashitaba has substantial levels of vitamin B12 and chalconoids that are unique to this species of angelica.

Chalconoids, also known as chalcones, are natural phenols related to chalcone. They show antibacterial, antifungal, antitumor and anti-inflammatory properties. Chalcones are also natural aromatase inhibitors.

Astragulus

Astragalus propinquus (syn. Astragalus membranaceus), is a flowering plant in the family Fabaceae.

Astragalus propinquus contains the saponin cycloastragenol. Constituents of the roots (Radix Astragali) include polysaccharides, triterpenoids (astragalosides) as well as isoflavones (including kumatakenin, calycosin and formononetin) along with their glycosides and malonates.

Cistanche

Cistanche tubulosa is a holoparasitic desert plant species in the genus Cistanche.

Cistanche tubulosa shows action in upregulating nerve growth factor.

Codonopsis pilosula

Codonopsis pilosula, also known as dang shen or poor man's ginseng, is a perennial species of flowering plant in the bellflower family.

Codonopsis pilosula has many pharmacological actions:

It regulates gastrointestinal motility, fight against ulcer, and enhance immunity;

It affects both excitatory and inhibitory neural processes;

Saponins of Codonopsis excite the respiratory center;

It lowers the animal blood pressure temporarily but raises the blood pressure on rabbits that are in late hemorrhagic shock;

It significantly increases rabbits' blood sugar. And rise of serum glucose level is related to the sugar contained;

It increases animal erythrocytes, hemoglobin, and reticulocytes;

It also delays aging, and fights anoxia and radiation.

Gastrodia elata (Gastrodin)

Gastrodia elata is a saprophytic perennial herb of the Orchidaceae family.

Gastrodia elata contains 4-Hydroxybenzaldehyde and gastrodin.   It also produces 2,4-Bis(4-hydroxybenzyl) phenol, gastrol, gast rodigenin and other related compounds.

Ginkgo Biloba

Ginkgo Biloba, also known as the maidenhair tree, is a unique species of tree and is the only extant taxon in the division Ginkgophyta. The ginkgo is a living fossil, recognisably similar to fossils dating back 270 million years.

Gotu Kola

Centella asiatica, commonly known as centella and gotu kola, is a small, herbaceous, annual plant of the family Mackinlayaceae or subfamily Mackinlayoideae of family Apiaceae, and is native to wetlands in Asia.

Centella asiatica has large amounts of pentacyclic triterpenoids including asiaticoside, brahmoside, asiatic acid, and brahmic acid also known as madecassic acid. Other products include centellose, centelloside, and madecassoside.

Green Tea

Green tea is made from the leaves from Camellia sinensis that have undergone minimal oxidation during processing.

Green tea contains favonols or flavanols.   The flavanols are comprised of catechins. There are four main classifications of catechins:

> epigallocatechin-3-gallate (EGCG)

> epi-gallocatechin (EGC)

> epicatechin gallate (ECG)

> epicatechin (EC)

Epigallocatechin-3-gallate (EGCG) is the most potent of the four catechins.

Gynostemma pentaphyllum (Jiaogulan)

Gynostemma pentaphyllum, also called jiaogulan is a dioecious, herbaceous climbing vine of the family Cucurbitaceae.

In China it is called the "immortality herb", since the people of the Guizhou Province, where jiaogulan herbal teas are consumed regularly, are said to have a history of unusual longevity.

Korean Ginseng

Ginsengs are plants from the Panax species of the Aralia (Araliaceae) family that possess very similar beneficial actions.

There are over 12 species of ginseng but five are used medicinally.   These five ginsengs include:

> Korean Ginseng (Panax Ginseng)

American Ginseng (Panax quinquefolius, aka Xiyangshen)

Vietnamese Ginseng (Panax vietnamensis)

Japanese Ginseng (Panax Japonicus)

Pseudoginseng or Sanchi Ginseng (Panax Notoginseng)

Of the five ginsengs, Korean Ginseng or Panax Ginseng is the most commonly used species medicinally.

Palmitine

Palmatine is a protoberberine alkaloid found in several plants. Palmatine a naturally existing alkaloid isolated from a medicinal plant Tinospora cordifolia.

Polygala teniufolia

Polygala tenuifolia (Yuan Zhi) is an herb in the family Polygalaceae.

Polygala tenuifolia has demonstrated potent and extensive neuroprotection benefits.   Studies have concluded that Polygala teniufolia tested in in healthy adults produced:

Memory-enhancing effects

Cognitive improvement

Increases NGF secretion in astrocytes

Potent antidepressant-like effects

Inhibited MAO-A and MAO-B activity,

Blocked stress-induced elevations of plasma cortisol

Improved hippocampal-dependent learning and memory

Rescued stress-induced deficits in hippocampal neuronal plasticity and neurogenesis

Displays anti-inflammatory activity towards microglia

Rehmannia

Rehmannia is a genus of six species of flowering plants in the order Lamiales.

Rehmannia contains compounds such as catalpol. Catalpol is known to exert protective effects on dopaminergic neurons reducing the production of pro-inflammatory factors.

Rosemary

Rosmarinus officinalis, commonly known as rosemary, is a woody, perennial herb with fragrant, evergreen, needle-like leaves and white, pink, purple, or blue flowers, native to the Mediterranean region. It is a member of the mint family Lamiaceae.

Rosemary contains carnosic acid, that is able to fight off free radical damage in the brain.

Rosemary contains a number of phytochemicals, including rosmarinic acid, camphor, caffeic acid, ursolic acid and betulinic acid.

Hormones

Melatonin

Melatonin is a hormone synthesized from the amino acid tryptophan. Melatonin controls the daily night-day cycle, thereby allowing the entrainment of the circadian rhythms of several biological functions. the other biological role of Melatonin is that of a powerful antioxidant.

Pregnenolone

Pregnenolone is an endogenous steroid hormone. It is the precursor of the progestogens, mineralocorticoids, glucocorticoids, androgens, and estrogens, as well as the neuroactive steroids. Pregnenolone also acts as a neurosteroid.

Neurosteroids affect synaptic functioning, are neuroprotective, and enhance myelinization.

Irisin

FNDC5 was initially discovered in 2002 during a genome search for fibronectin type III domains and also independently in a search for peroxisomal proteins.

Irisin is a protein that in humans is encoded by the FNDC5 gene.

Krebs Cycle Chemicals

Oxaloacetate (Oxaloacetic Acid)

Oxaloacetic acid is a metabolic intermediate in many biological processes, including: gluconeogenesis, urea cycle, glyoxylate cycle, amino acid synthesis, fatty acid synthesis and citric acid cycle.

Oxaloacetate is a natural energy molecule that is critical to human metabolism and proper cellular function. Oxaloacetic Acid is a type of dicarboxylic acid that is one of the endogenous chemicals involved in the Krebs Cycle of endogenous energy production.

Oxaloacetate is a bio-identical human metabolite that increases the NAD+/NADH ratio, and has been proven to result a 25% increase in lifespan in laboratory animals ($p < 0.001$).

Lipids

Queen Bee Acid (Royal Jelly) (10-hydroxy-2-decenoic acid)

Queen Bee Acid (Royal Jelly) (10-hydroxy-2-decenoic acid) is a bio-active compound found in royal jelly.

Myrmicacin (3-hydroxydecanoic acid) is also found in royal jelly. 10-Hydroxydecanic acid is a specialized unsaturated fatty acid that is a constituent of royal jelly and bee pollen.

Queen bee acid has similar neurogenic effects in animal and in vitro tests to the omega 3 fatty acid docosahexaenoic acid (DHA) and the protein brain-derived neurotrophic factor (BDNF).

Queen bee acid activates AMP-activated protein kinase (AMPK) and enhances glucose uptake.

Docosahexaenoic acid (DHA)

Docosahexaenoic acid (DHA) is an omega-3 fatty acid that is a primary structural component of the human brain, cerebral cortex, skin, sperm, testicles and retina. It can be synthesized from alpha-linolenic acid or obtained directly from maternal milk or fish oil.

More than two thirds of the dry weight of the human brain is fat, and of that fat, one quarter is docosahexaenoic acid (DHA).   DHA is an important building block for the membranes surrounding brain cells, particulary the synapses, which lie at the heart of efficient brain function.

DHA also regulates the production of Brain Derived Neurotrophic Factor (BDNF). DHA orchestrates the production, connectivity, and vialbility of brain cells while at the same time enhancing function.

In healthy people, DHA brain uptake is 4 mg per day and ARA is 18 mg per day. There are 5 grams of DHA in the brain. If decreased by a third, it would take a year to bring it back to the normal level.

Phosphatidylserine

Phosphatidylserine is a phospholipid cell membrane component which plays a key role in cell cycle signaling.   Half the bodys phosphatidylserine storage (60g) is found in the neural tissue.

Minerals

Magnesiun-l-threonate (Magtein (TM))

Magnesiun-l-threonate consists of magnesium bonded to the organic acid, threonic acid, and is denoted by the chemical formula $Mg(C_4H_7O_5)_2$.

Magnesiun-l-threonate has high brain bioavailability. It is the only magnesium compound that has been shown to effectively raise the brain's magnesium levels.

In pre-clinical models, L-threonate contained in Magnesiun-l-threonate boosted magnesium levels in spinal fluid by an impressive 15% compared to no increase with conventional magnesium.

Research on Magnesiun-l-threonate has been led by the biopharmaceutical company Magceutics of Hayward, California.   They tradmarked the product named Magtein(TM).   They began testing Magtein,'s(TM) ability to boost magnesium ion ($Mg2+$) levels in the brain in 2012 and the results have been impressive.

Lithium (Lithium Orotate)

Lithium orotate, is a salt of orotic acid and lithium.

It is used in small doses to treat certain medical conditions, such as stress, bipolar disorder, depression, suicidal ideations, alcoholism, ADHD, attention deficit disorder, aggression, PTSD, Alzheimer's and to improve memory.

Nootropics

Deprenyl

Selegiline (Anipryl, L-deprenyl, Eldepryl, Emsam, Zelapar) is a drug used for the treatment of early-stage Parkinson's disease, depression and dementia. In normal clinical doses it is a selective irreversible MAO-B inhibitor.

The drug was discovered by József Knoll et al. in Hungary.   It was developed specifically as a nootropic. It was developed as a way to study high-performing individuals, and seeing if it was possible to replicate those through pharmaceuticals.

It requires a physician's prescription in the U.S., but may be bought without a prescription from an offshore pharmacy.

Galantamine

Galantamine is an alkaloid that is obtained synthetically or from the bulbs and flowers of Galanthus caucasicus (Caucasian snowdrop, Voronov's snowdrop), Galanthus woronowii (Amaryllidaceae) and related genera like Narcissus (daffodil), Leucojum (snowflake), and Lycoris including Lycoris radiata (Red Spider Lily).

It is used for the treatment of mild to moderate Alzheimer's disease and various other memory impairments, in particular those of vascular origin.

Hydergine

Ergoloid mesylates (USAN), co-dergocrine mesilate (BAN) or dihydroergotoxine mesylate, trade name Hydergine, is a mixture of the methanesulfonate salts of three dihydrogenated ergot alkaloids (dihydroergocristine, dihydroergocornine, and alpha- and beta-dihydroergocryptine).

It was developed by Albert Hofmann (the inventor of LSD) for Sandoz (now part of Novartis).

It has been used to treat dementia and age-related cognitive impairment (such as in Alzheimer disease), as well as to aid in recovery after stroke.

There is some evidence suggesting that potentially effective doses may be higher than those currently approved in dementia treatment.

It requires a physician's prescription in the U.S., but may be bought without a prescription from an offshore pharmacy.

Idebenone

Idebenone (full structural name of 6-(10-hydroxydecyl)-2,3-dimethoxy-5-methyl-1,4-benzoquinone and codename of-2619[1]) is a synthetic derivative of ubiquinone (reduced CoQ10).

COQ10 is a long chained compound while Idebenone is a short chained compound. This means that idebenone has a much higher level of bioavailability than CoQ10.

Like its parent compound, it is a powerful antioxidant with additional nootropic benefits including improving memory, learning, and symptoms of age related memory loss. Idebenone is also able to increase adenosine triphosphate (ATP) production.

It also provides a basic level of neuroprotection and is a mood booster since it is able to boost dopamine levels within the brain.

Nicergoline

Nicergoline (INN, marketed under the trade name Sermion) is an ergot derivative used to treat senile dementia and other disorders with vascular origins. It has been found to increase mental agility and enhance clarity and perception. It decreases vascular resistance and increases arterial blood flow in the brain, improving the utilization of oxygen and glucose by brain cells. It has similar vasoactive properties in other areas of the body, particularly the lungs.

Nicergoline is an ergot alkaloid derivative that acts as a potent and selective alpha-1A adrenergic receptor antagonist.

It requires a physician's prescription in the U.S., but may be bought without a prescription from an offshore pharmacy.

Noopept

Noopept (Russian: Ноопепт; GVS-111, N-phenylacetyl-L-prolylglycine ethyl ester) is a peptide promoted and prescribed in Russia and neighbouring countries as a nootropic. The registered brand name Noopept (Ноопепт) is trademarked by the manufacturer JSC LEKKO Pharmaceuticals. The compound is patented in both the US and Russia with patent of Russian Federation number 2119496, US Patent number 5,439,930 issued 8/8/1995.

Noopept is in effect to Piracetam and is often cited as being 1000 times more potent (by weight) than Piracetam. Noopept has high oral bioavailability.

Semax

Semax is a drug produced and prescribed mostly in Russia and Ukraine for a broad range of conditions but predominantly for its purported nootropic, neuroprotective, and neurogenic/neurorestorative properties.

It is a heptapeptide, synthetic analog of a fragment of adrenocorticotropic hormone (ACTH), ACTH (4-10), of the following structure: Met-Glu-His-Phe-Pro-Gly-Pro. Semax has not been evaluated by the U.S. FDA. It is unscheduled in the U.S. and legal to import by private citizens for personal use.

In Russia, Semax is used to treat stroke, brain damage following ischemia, optic nerve disease and as a treatment for various cognitive disorders.

In glial cell cultures, both BDNF and NGF levels were increased 8 fold and 5 fold following exposure to Semax . In rodents, Semax has been shown to increase BDNF and trkB levels by 1.4 and 1.6 fold respectively. Further research has shown intranasal administration of Semax is able to increase BDNF in the rat brain.

Nucelic Compounds

Uridine-5'-monophosphate (UMP)

Uridine-5'-monophosphate is a nucleotide that is used as a monomer in RNA. It is an ester of phosphoric acid with the nucleoside uridine. Uridine is one of the building blocks or precursor components to Ribonucleic Acid (RNA).

UMP supplementation stimulates the production of neurotransmitters and neurites.

Triacetyluridine (TAU)

Triacetyluridine (TAU) is a prodrug of uridine, meaning it is a more bio available form.   It is rapidly converted within the body to Uridine.   TAU has 7-fold greater bioavailability than an equimolar amount of Uridine.

TAU is able to enhance nerve growth factor (NGF) by activating P2Y2 receptors within the brain, thus increasing neuron growth.

Polyphenols

Quercetin

Quercetin is a flavonol found in many fruits, vegetables, leaves and grains.

Quercetin is found mostly in onions and grapes.

Curcumin

Curcumin is a diarylheptanoid. It is the principal curcuminoid of turmeric, which is a member of the ginger family (Zingiberaceae). Turmeric's other two curcuminoids are desmethoxycurcumin and bis-desmethoxycurcumin. The curcuminoids are natural phenols that are responsible for the yellow color of turmeric.

7,8-dihydroxyflavone (7,8-DHF)

7,8-Dihydroxyflavone (7,8-DHF) is a synthetic flavone derivative. It is a potent and selective agonist of the TrkB receptor, which is the main signaling receptor of brain-derived neurotrophic factor (BDNF).   It is able to penetrate the blood-brain-barrier and thus is bio-available.

7,8-DHF has been very therapeutically efficient in various central nervous system disorders including:

Depression
Alzheimer's disease
Schizophrenia
Parkinson's disease
Huntington's disease
Amyotrophic lateral sclerosis
Traumatic brain injury
Cerebral ischemia

Proteins

Lactoferrin

Lactoferrin (LF), also known as lactotransferrin (LTF), is a multifunctional protein of the transferrin family.

Lactoferrin is one of the components of the immune system of the body; it has antimicrobial activity (bacteriocide, fungicide) and is part of the innate defense, mainly at mucoses.

Quinones

Pyrroloquinoline Quinone

Pyrroloquinoline quinone (PQQ) is the third redox cofactor after nicotinamide and flavin in bacteria.

PQQ is a neuroprotective compound that has been shown in a small number of preliminary studies to protect memory and cognition in humans.

Spices

Ceylon Cinnamon (True Cinnamon)

Cinnamon is a spice obtained from the inner bark of several trees from the genus Cinnamomum that is used in both sweet and savoury foods. Cinnamomum verum is considered to be "true cinnamon" versus a related species, referred to as "Cinnamomum cassia".   It is the true cinnamon (Cinnamomum verum) that is referred to in this text.

Cinnamon contains a number of bioactive substances:

> Cinnamaldehydes
>
> Coumarins (a toxin) contribute to taste
>
> MethylHydroxyChalcone polymers (MHCPs)
>
> Tannins
>
> Flavonoids
>
> Glycosides
>
> Terpenoids
>
> Anthraquinones

Tumeric

Turmeric (Curcuma longa) is a rhizomatous herbaceous perennial plant of the ginger family, Zingiberaceae.

The most important chemical components of turmeric are a group of compounds called curcuminoids, which include curcumin (diferuloylmethane), demethoxycurcumin, and bisdemethoxycurcumin. The best-studied compound is curcumin, which constitutes 3.14% (on average) of powdered turmeric.   In addition, other important volatile oils include turmerone ar=tumerone, atlantone, and zingiberene.

Sage (Salvia officinalis)

Salvia officinalis (sage, also called garden sage, or common sage) is a perennial, evergreen subshrub. It is a member of the family Lamiaceae and is native to the Mediterranean region.   Researchers concluded that extracts of sage can enhance cognitive performance.

Vitamins

Vitamin B5 (Pantethine form)

Pantethine is a highly absorbable and biologically active form of Pantothenic Acid (Vitamin B-5). The metabolic activity of Pantethine is due to its role in the formation of Coenzyme A (CoA), an essential cofactor for lipid, carbohydrate, and protein metabolism.

Alpha-GPC

Alpha GPC is a naturally occurring choline intermediary that is formed when the body breaks down cell membranes for choline.

Alpha-GPC is a form of choline that consists of Choline bound to Glycerophosphate.   It is the most bioavailable form of Choline.   It is more potent than other forms of Choline (including Cytidine Diphosphate Choline (CDP-Choline)).

As a supplement Alpha GPC is a highly bio available form of choline that crosses the blood brain barrier and raises brain levels of choline.

Appendix B: Sources for Products and Substances

Table 5.1 provides a number of sources for the more uncommon and esoteric substances in this book. Those substances not listed in Table 5.1 can be purchased at your local health food store.

Table 5.1 Sources for Products and Substances

Sources		
Catagory	**Product/Substance**	**Source/Resource**
Alkaloids		
	Berberine	Thorne Research Piping Rock Integrative Theraputics Nutriguard Research
	Huperzine A	Source Naturals Solaray Swansons Nature's Plus
Amino acids		
	L-Theanine	Swansons Now Source Naturals
	Beta-Alanine	Pure Bulk (powder and capsules) Powder City (powder) Swansons (powder) Bodystrong (powder)
	Acetyl-L-Carnitine (ALCAR)	Pure Bulk (powder) Powder City (powder) Jarrow Life Extension Swansons
	Taurine	Pure Bulk (powder) Jarrow Formula's Life Extension
	Proline-rich polypeptide	Symbiotic's (powder)
Foods		

	Grape Seed Extract	Pure Bulk (powder extract) Food Science of Vermont Now Nature's Way
	Euphoria Longan (fruit/berry)	Swansons Chinese Herbs Direct Jing Herbs Dragon Herbs (fruit)
	Cacao	Navitas Naturals (powder, nibs, beans) Sunfood (powder, nibs, beans)
	Blueberries	Fresh and frozen Nuts.com (powder extract) LiveSuperfoods (powder extract)
Fungi		
	Lions Mane	Host Defense Mushroom Science Paradise Herbs
Herbs		
	Ahwagandha	Ojio (powder) Jarrow Sun Portion (powder)
	Gotu Kola	Nature's Way Swansons Starwest Botanicals
	Gynostemma pentaphyllum (Jiaogulan)	Paradise Herbs Planetary Herbals Om-Chi Herbs Max Nature
	Cistanche	Jing Herbs (powder) Life Extension Barlowe's Herbal Elixirs
	Codonopsis pilosula	HerBulk (bulk herb) Chinese Herbs Direct (extract) Om-Chi Herbs Max Nature
	Ginko Biloba	Jarrow Doctor's Best

		Max Nature
	Polygala teniufolia	Plum Flower Brand Stakich Herbal Extracts ThebestEver (eBay) (powder) Om-Chi Herbs Max Nature
	Astragulus	Swansons Gaia Herbs Paradice Herbs
	Green Tea	Green Foods (Matcha powder) Jarrow
	Gastrodia elata (Gastrodin)	Life Extension Om-Chi Herbs Max Nature
	Rosemary	Nature's Way Solaray Starwest Botanicals (leaf) Frontier Natural Products (leaf)
	Rehmannia	Planetary Herbals Bulk Apothecary (root) Herb Pharm (liquid extract) Health Concerns
	Korean Ginseng	Swansons Imperial Elixir Max Nature
	Ashitaba (Angelica keiskei)	Percent Ashitaba Swansons Sun Portion (powder)
	Palmitine (Tinospora cordifolia (Guduchi))	Life Extension Himalaya Herbal Healthcare Banyan Botanicals (powder) Max Nature
Hormones		
	Pregnenolone	Swansons Life Extension Ortho Molecular Products
	Melatonin	Life Extension (fast acting liquid) Source Naturals (sublingual)

	Irisin	Not available at time of publication. Contact health care provider.
Krebs Cycle Chemicals		
	Oxaloacetate	Benegene Bulletproof
Lipids		
	(Docosahexaenoic acid (DHA))	Carlson Labs Nordic Naturals Premier Research Labs Doctors Best
	Queen Bee Acid (Royal Jelly)	Antaeus Labs
	Royal Jelly	Immortality's Alchemy
	Phosphatidylserine	Swansons Jarrow Solgar
Minerals		
	Magnesiun-l-threonate (Magtein (TM))	Life Extension (capsules and powder) Source Natruals Doctor's Best Jarrow
	Lithium (Lithium Orotate)	NutrientCarriers KAL Ortho Molecular Products
Nootropics		
	Deprenyl	International Anti-Aging Systems (Offshore Pharmacy)
	Hydergine	International Anti-Aging Systems (Offshore Pharmacy)
	Nicergoline	International Anti-Aging Systems (Offshore Pharmacy)
	Idebenone	Relentless Improvement Powder City

		Kirkman Labs
	Galantamine	Antaeus Labs Life Enhancement Relentless Improvement
	Semax	Ceretropic (U.S.) SmartNootropics (U.K./Europe)
	Noopept	CTD Labs Relentless Improvement Cognitive Nutrition Peak Nootropics Pure Nootropics (sublingual) Powder City
Nucelic Compounds		
	Uridine-5'-monophosphate	Jarrow Cardiovascular Research Ltd. Bonanza (online powder)
	Triacetyluridine (TAU)	Powder City (powder) Antaeus Labs
Polyphenols		
	Quercetin	Jarrow Swansons
	Curcumin	Life Extension (BCM-95(TM)) Empircal Labs (liposomal curcumin) MaxHealthLabs (liposomal) Powder City (tumeric extract 95%) Swanson (Theracurmin(TM)) Source Naturals (Meriva(TM))
	7,8-dihydroxyflavone (7,8-DHF)	Antaleus Labs Lockout Supplements Primordial Muscle
Proteins		
	Lactoferrin	Swansons Jarrow Life Extension
Quinones		

	Pyrroloquinoline Quinone	Life Extension Jarrow Doctor's Best Swansons
Spices		
	Ceylon Cinnamon	Savory Spice Shop (powder) My Spice Sage (powder) The Spice House (powder) Carlson's Labs (capsules)
	Tumeric	Roots can be bought at ethnic markets (Asian, Persian, Indian) Powder City (Tumeric powder)
Vitamins		
	Vitamin B5 (Pantethine form)	Jarrow Swansons
	Alpha-GPC	Jarrow Swansons Powder City (powder)

Endnotes/References

[1] http://www.nature.com/nm/journal/v4/n11/full/nm1198_1313.html

[2] http://www.nature.com/nm/journal/v4/n11/abs/nm1198_1313.html

[3] Spalding KL, Bergmann O, Alkass K, Bernard S, Salehpour M, Huttner HB, Boström E, Westerlund I, Vial C, Buchholz BA, Possnert G, Mash DC, Druid H, Frisén J. Dynamics of hippocampal neurogenesis in adult humans. *Cell.* 2013 Jun 6;153(6):1219-27.

[4] Gould, E.; Reeves, A. J.; Graziano, M. S.; Gross, C. G. (1999). "Neurogenesis in the neocortex of adult primates". *Science* **286** (5439): 548–552. doi:10.1126/science.286.5439.548. PMID 10521353.

Zhao, M.; Momma, S.; Delfani, K.; Carlen, M.; Cassidy, R. M.; Johansson, C. B.; Brismar, H.; Shupliakov, O.; Frisen, J.; Janson, A. (2003). "Evidence for neurogenesis in the adult mammalian substantia nigra". *Proceedings of the National Academy of Sciences of the United States of America* **100** (13): 7925–7930. Bibcode:2003PNAS..100.7925Z. doi:10.1073/pnas.1131955100. PMC 164689. PMID 12792021.

Shankle; Rafii, M. S.; Landing, B. H.; Fallon, J. H. (1999). "Approximate doubling of numbers of neurons in postnatal human cerebral cortex and in 35 specific cytoarchitectural areas from birth to 72 months". *Pediatric and developmental pathology : the official journal of the Society for Pediatric Pathology and the Paediatric Pathology Society* **2** (3): 244–259. doi:10.1007/s100249900120. PMID 10191348

[5] Prull MW, Gabrieli JDE, Bunge SA (2000). "Ch 2. Age-related changes in memory: A cognitive neuroscience perspective". In Craik FIM, Salthouse TA. *The handbook of aging and cognition.* Erlbaum. ISBN 978-0-8058-2966-2.

[6] D. C. Lie, H. Song, S. A. Colamarino, G. L. Ming, and F. H. Gage, "Neurogenesis in the adult brain: new strategies for central nervous system diseases," *Annual Review of Pharmacology and Toxicology,* vol. 44, pp. 399–421, 2004.

C. Mirescu and E. Gould, "Stress and adult neurogenesis," *Hippocampus,* vol. 16, no. 3, pp. 233–238, 2006.

A. Sahay and R. Hen, "Adult hippocampal neurogenesis in depression," *Nature Neuroscience,* vol. 10, no. 9, pp. 1110–1115, 2007.

[7] Lemaire, V., Tronel, S., Montaron, M. F., Fabre, A., Dugast, E., and Abrous, D. N. (2012). Long-lasting plasticity of hippocampal adult-born neurons. *J. Neurosci.* 32, 3101–3108. doi: 10.1523/JNEUROSCI.4731-11.2012

[8] G. Neves, G; S.F. Cooke and T.V. Bliss (2008). "Synaptic plasticity, memory and the hippocampus: A neural network approach to causality". *Nature Reviews Neuroscience* **9** (1): 65–75. doi:10.1038/nrn2303. PMID 18094707.

Becker S (2005). "A computational principle for hippocampal learning and neurogenesis". *Hippocampus* **15** (6): 722–38. doi:10.1002/hipo.20095. PMID 15986407.

Wiskott L, Rasch MJ, Kempermann G (2006). "A functional hypothesis for adult hippocampal neurogenesis: avoidance of catastrophic interference in the dentate gyrus". *Hippocampus* **16** (3): 329–43. doi:10.1002/hipo.20167. PMID 16435309.

Aimone JB, Wiles J, Gage FH (June 2006). "Potential role for adult neurogenesis in the encoding of time in new memories". *Nat Neurosci.* **9** (6): 723–7. doi:10.1038/nn1707. PMID 16732202

[9] Shors TJ, Townsend DA, Zhao M, Kozorovitskiy Y, Gould E (2002). "Neurogenesis may relate to some but not all types of hippocampal-dependent learning". *Hippocampus* **12** (5): 578–84. doi:10.1002/hipo.10103. PMC 3289536. PMID 12440573.

Meshi D, Drew MR, Saxe M, et al. (June 2006). "Hippocampal neurogenesis is not required for behavioral effects of environmental enrichment". *Nat Neurosci.* **9** (6): 729–31. doi:10.1038/nn1696. PMID 16648847.

Gould, E.; Beylin, A.; Tanapat, P.; Reeves, A.; Shors, T. J. (1999). "Learning enhances adult neurogenesis in the hippocampal formation". *Nature Neuroscience* **2** (3): 260–265. doi:10.1038/6365. PMID 10195219.

[10] Donovan, M. H.; Yazdani, U; Norris, R. D.; Games, D; German, D. C.; Eisch, A. J. (2006). "Decreased adult hippocampal neurogenesis in the PDAPP mouse model of Alzheimer's disease". *The Journal of Comparative Neurology* **495** (1): 70–83. doi:10.1002/cne.20840. PMID 16432899.

[11] Jacobs, B. L., H. van Praag, F. H. Gage (2000). "Depression and the Birth and Death of Brain Cells". *American Scientist* **88**.

Kandel, E. R., J. H. Schwartz and T. M. Jessell (2012-10-26). *Principles of Neural Science, fifth edition.* ISBN 0071390111.

[12] Schloesser RJ, Manji HK, Martinowich K (April 2009). "Suppression of adult neurogenesis leads to an increased hypothalamo-pituitary-adrenal axis response.". *NeuroReport* **20** (6): 553–7. doi:10.1097/WNR.0b013e3283293e59. PMC 2693911. PMID 19322118.

Surget A, Tanti A, Leonardo ED et al. (December 2011). "Antidepressants recruit new neurons to improve stress response regulation.". *Molecular Psychiatry* **16** (12): 1177–88. doi:10.1038/mp.2011.48. PMC 3223314. PMID 21537331.

[13] Wentz CT, Magavi SSP (2009) Caffeine alters proliferation of neuronal precursors in the adult hippocampus. Neuropharmacology 56(6–7):994–1000

[14] Nixon K, Crews FT (2002) Binge ethanol exposure decreases neurogenesis in adult rat hippocampus. J Neurochem 83:1087–1093

He J, Nixon K, Shetty AK, Crews FT (2005) Chronic alcohol exposure reduces hippocampal neurogenesis and dendritic growth of newborn neurons. Eur J Neurosci 21:2711–2720

Stevenson JR, Schroeder JP, Nixon K, Besheer J, Crews FT, Hodge CW (2008) Abstinence following alcohol drinking produces depression-like behavior and reduced hippocampal neurogenesis in mice. Neuropsychopharmacology 34:1209–1222

[15] Lindqvist A, Mohapel P, Bouter B, Frielingsdorf H, Pizzo D, Brundin P, Erlanson-Albertsson C (2006) High-fat diet impairs hippocampal neurogenesis in male rats. Eur J Neurol 13:1385–1388

[16] Rabaneda LG, Carrasco M, Lopez-Toledano MA, Murillo-Carretero M, Ruiz FA, Estrada C, Castro C (2008) Homocysteine inhibits proliferation of neuronal precursors in the mouse adult brain by impairing the basic fibroblast growth factor signaling cascade and r

[17] Molteni, R., et al. A high-fat, refined sugar diet reduces hippocampal brain-derived neurotrophic factor, neuronal plasticity, and learning. Neuroscience. 112(4):803-814, 2002.

Wu, A., et al. A saturated-fat diet aggravates the outcome of traumatic brain injury on hippocampal plasticity and cognitive function by reducing brain-derived neurotrophic factor. Neuroscience. 119(2):365-375, 2003.

[18] http://neuronalsurvival.se/wp-content/uploads/2008/10/van_der_broght-2010-regl.pept.pdf

[19] Lee AL, Ogle WO, Sapolsky RM (April 2002). "Stress and depression: possible links to neuron death in the hippocampus". *Bipolar Disord.* **4** (2): 117–28. doi:10.1034/j.1399-5618.2002.01144.x. PMID 12071509.

[20] Sheline YI, Gado MH, Kraemer HC (August 2003). "Untreated depression and hippocampal volume loss". *Am J Psychiatry.* **160** (8): 1516–8. doi:10.1176/appi.ajp.160.8.1516. PMID 12900317.

[21] Mirescu C, Peters JD, Noiman L, Gould E (December 2006). "Sleep deprivation inhibits adult neurogenesis in the hippocampus by elevating glucocorticoids". *Proc. Natl. Acad. Sci. U.S.A.* **103** (50): 19170–5. Bibcode:2006PNAS..10319170M. doi:10.1073/pnas.0608644103. PMC 1748194. PMID 17135354.

C. Mirescu, J. D. Peters, L. Noiman, E. Gould: *Sleep deprivation inhibits adult neurogenesis in the hippocampus by elevating glucocorticoids.* In: *Proceedings of the National Academy of Sciences.* 103, 2006, p. 19170–19175, doi:10.1073/pnas.0608644103.

[22] The Intestinal Microbiota Affect Central Levels of Brain-Derived Neurotropic Factor and Behavior in Mice

[23] Antenatal taurine supplementation improves cerebral neurogenesis in fetal rats with intrauterine growth restriction through the PKA-CREB signal pathway.

Ripps, Shen. Review: Taurine: a 'very essential' amino acid. *Mol Vis.* 18:2673-86 (2012).

[24] Colostral proline-rich polypeptides--immunoregulatory properties and prospects of therapeutic use in Alzheimer's disease.

[25] Grape seed extract enhances neurogenesis in the hippocampal dentate gyrus in C57BL/6 mice.

[26] Casadesus G, Shukitt-Hale B, Stellwagen HM, Zhu X, Lee HG, Smith MA, Joseph JA (2004) Modulation of hippocampal plasticity and cognitive behavior by short-term blueberry supplementation in aged rats. Nutr Neurosci 7:309–316

[27] Tohda C, Kuboyama T, Komatsu K. Search for natural products related to regeneration of the neuronal network. *Neurosignals.* (2005)

Kuboyama T, *et al.* Axon- or dendrite-predominant outgrowth induced by constituents from Ashwagandha. *Neuroreport.* (2002)

Kuboyama T, Tohda C, Komatsu K. Neuritic regeneration and synaptic reconstruction induced by withanolide A. *Br J Pharmacol.* (2005) J

ana CK, *et al.* Synthesis of withanolide A, biological evaluation of its neuritogenic properties, and studies on secretase inhibition. *Angew Chem Int Ed Engl.* (2011)

Tohda C, Kuboyama T, Komatsu K. Dendrite extension by methanol extract of Ashwagandha (roots of Withania somnifera) in SK-N-SH cells. *Neuroreport.* (2000)

Tohda C, Joyashiki E. Sominone enhances neurite outgrowth and spatial memory mediated by the neurotrophic factor receptor, RET. *Br J Pharmacol.* (2009)

Kuboyama T, Tohda C, Komatsu K. Withanoside IV and its active metabolite, sominone, attenuate Abeta(25-35)-induced neurodegeneration. *Eur J Neurosci.* (2006)

Withanoside IV and its active metabolite, sominone, attenuate Aβ(25–35)-induced neurodegeneration

[28] Green tea epigallocatechin-3-gallate (EGCG) promotes neural progenitor cell proliferation and sonic hedgehog pathway activation during adult hippocampal neurogenesis.

[29] Ramachandran U, Manavalan A, Sundaramurthi H, et al. Tianma modulates proteins with various neuro-regenerative modalities in differentiated human neuronal SH-SY5Y cells. *Neurochem Int.* 2012 Jun;60(8):827-36.

Manavalan A, Ramachandran U, Sundaramurthi H, et al. Gastrodia elata Blume (tianma) mobilizes neuro-protective capacities. *Int J Biochem Mol Biol.* 2012;3(2):219-41.

[30] Cannabinoids promote embryonic and adult hippocampus neurogenesis and produce anxiolytic- and antidepressant-like effectsWen Jiang[1,2], Yun Zhang[1], Lan Xiao[1], Jamie Van Cleemput[1], Shao-Ping Ji[1], Guang Bai[3] and Xia Zhang[1]

[31] http://www.jneurosci.org/content/33/7/2961.full

[32] Pregnenolone sulfate enhances neurogenesis and PSA-NCAM in young and aged hippocampus.

Mayo W, Lemaire V, Malaterre J, et al. Pregnenolone sulfate enhances neurogenesis and PSA-NCAM in young and aged hippocampus. Neurobiol Aging. 2005 Jan;26(1):103-14.

Mayo W, George O, Darbra S, et al. Individual differences in cognitive aging: implication of pregnenolone sulfate. Prog Neurobiol. 2003 Sep;71(1):43-8.

[33] Effects of melatonin on nervous system aging: neurogenesis and neurodegeneration.

[34] IMPACT OF OXALOACETATE ON BRAIN BIOENERGETIC INFRASTRUCTURES, NEUROGENESIS, AND INFLAMMATION

[35] Omega-3 fatty acids upregulate adult neurogenesis.

n-3 fatty acids: role in neurogenesis and neuroplasticity.

[36] Improved spatial learning performance of fat-1 mice is associated with enhanced neurogenesis and neuritogenesis by docosahexaenoic acid

[37] Kawakita E, Hashimoto M, Shido O (2006) Docosahexaenoic acid promotes neurogenesis in vitro and in vivo. Neuroscience 139:991–997

[38] Royal Jelly and Its Unique Fatty Acid, 10-Hydroxy-Trans-2-Decenoic Acid, Promote Neurogenesis by Neural Stem/progenitor Cells in Vitro. Biomedical Research (Tokyo, Japan) 28(5): 261–266.

[39] Zinc and Neurogenesis: Making New Neurons from Development to Adulthood, doi: 10.3945/ an.110.000174   Adv Nutr March 2011   Adv Nutr   vol. 2:   96-100,   2011

[40] Wada A, Yokoo H, Yanagita T, Kobayashi H. Lithium: potential therapeutics against acute brain injuries and chronic neurodegenerative diseases. *J Pharmacol Sci* 2005;99:307-21.

Moore GJ, Bebchuk JM, Wilds IB, Chen G, Manji HK. Lithium-induced increase in human brain grey matter. *Lancet* 2000;356(9237):1241-2. Erratum: *Lancet* 2000;356(9247):2104.

Moore GJ, Bebchuk JM, Hasanat K, Chen G, Seraji-Bozorgzad N, Wilds IB, Faulk MW, Koch S, Jolkovsky L, Manji HK. Lithium increases *N*-acetyl-aspartate in the human brain: in vivo evidence in support of bcl-2's neurotrophic effects? *Biol Psychiatry* 2000;48:1-8.

[41] Kita Y, Ago Y, Higashino K, Asada K, Takano E, Takuma K, Matsuda T. Galantamine promotes adult hippocampal neurogenesis via M1 muscarinic and α7 nicotinic receptors in mice. Int J *Neuropsychopharmacol.* 2014 May 12:1-12.

[42] Wang L, Pooler AM, Albrecht MA, Wurtman RJ. Dietary uridine-5'-monophosphate supplementation increases potassium-evoked dopamine release and promotes neurite outgrowth in aged rats. *J Mol Neurosci.* 2005;27(1):137-45.

[43] Curcumin Enhances Neurogenesis and Cognition in Aged Rats: Implications for Transcriptional Interactions Related to Growth and Synaptic Plasticity

[44] Kim SJ, Son TG, Park HR, Park M, Kim MS, Kim HS, Chung HY, Mattson MP, Lee J (2008) Curcumin stimulates proliferation of embryonic neural progenitor cells and neurogenesis in the adult hippocampus. J Biol Chem 283:14497–14505

[45] http://www.ncbi.nlm.nih.gov/pubmed/19441930

[46] Zhang L, Liu J, Cheng C, Yuan Y, Yu B, Shen A, Yan M. The neuroprotective effect of pyrroloquinoline quinone on traumatic brain injury. J Neurotrauma. 2012 Mar 20;29(5):851-64. Epub 2011 Dec 20.

[47] http://www.eurekalert.org/pub_releases/2014-09/bc-tcb092314.php

[48] Available at: http://informahealthcare.com/doi/abs/10.1517/13543770902721279. Accessed October 31, 2014.

[49] Zhao N, Zhong C, Wang Y, Zhao Y, Gong N, Zhou G, Xu T, Hong Z (2008) Impaired hippocampal neurogenesis is involved in cognitive dysfunction induced by thiamine deficiency at early pre-pathological lesion stage. Neurobiol Dis 29:176–185

[50] Folic acid enhances Notch signaling, hippocampal neurogenesis, and cognitive function in a rat model of cerebral ischemia.

[51] Kronenberg G, Harms C, Sobol RW, Cardozo-Pelaez F, Linhart H, Winter B, Balkaya M, Gertz K, Gay SB, Cox D, Eckart S, Ahmadi M, Juckel G, Kempermann G, Hellweg R, Sohr R, Hortnagl H, Wilson SH, Jaenisch R, Endres M (2008) Folate deficiency induces neurodege

Kruman II, Mouton PR, Emokpae R Jr, Cutler RG, Mattson MP (2005) Folate deficiency inhibits proliferation of adult hippocampal progenitors. Neuroreport 16:1055–1059

[52] A Mid-Life Vitamin A Supplementation Prevents Age-Related Spatial Memory Deficits and Hippocampal Neurogenesis Alterations through CRABP-I

[53] Bonnet E, Touyarot K, Alfos S, Pallet V, Higueret P, Abrous DN (2008) Retinoic acid restores adult hippocampal neurogenesis and reverses spatial memory deficit in vitamin A-deprived rats. PLoS ONE 3:e3487

[54] Rasmussen, P., et al. Evidence for a release of BDNF from the brain during exercise. Exp Physiol. 2009. University of Copenhagen;

Brain derived neurotrophic factor (BDNF) has an important role in regulating maintenance, growth and survival of neurons. However, the main source of circulating BDNF in response to exercise is unknown. To identify whether the brain is a source of BDNF during exercise, eight volunteers rowed for 4 hours while simultaneous blood samples were obtained from the radial artery and the internal jugular vein. To further identify putative cerebral region(s) responsible for BDNF release, mouse brains were dissected and analyzed for BDNF mRNA expression following treadmill exercise. In humans, a BDNF release from the brain was observed at rest (P < 0.05) and it increased 2-3 fold during exercise (P < 0.05).   Both at rest and during exercise, the brain contributed 70%-80% of circulating BDNF, while that contribution decreased following 1 hour of recovery.   In mice, exercise induced a 3-5 fold increase in BDNF mRNA expression in the hippocampus and cortex, peaking 2 hours after the termination of exercise.   These results suggest that the brain is a major but not sole contributor to circulating BDNF.   Moreover, the importance of the cortex and hippocampus as a source for plasma BDNF becomes even more prominent during exercise.

Strohle, A., et al.   Acute exercise ameliorates reduced brain-derived neurotrophic factor in patients with panic disorder.   Psychoneuroendocrinology.   2009.

The neurotrophin brain-derived neurotrophic factor (BDNF) has been implicated in depression and anxiety. Antidepressants and exercise increase BDNF expression, and both have an antidepressant and anxiolytic activity.   To further characterize the association of anxiety, BDNF and exercise, the authors studied panic disorder patients (n=12) and individually matched healthy control subjects (n=12) in a standardized exercise paradigm.   Serum samples for BDNF analyses were taken before and after 30min of exercise (70 VO(2max)) or quiet rest.   The two conditions were separated by 1 week and the order was randomized. Non-parametric statistical analyses were performed.   There was a negative correlation of BDNF concentrations and subjective arousal at baseline (r=-0.42, p=0.006).   Compared to healthy control subjects, patients with panic disorder had significantly reduced BDNF concentrations at baseline and 30 min of exercise significantly increased BDNF concentrations only in these patients.   These results suggest that acute exercise ameliorates reduced BDNF concentrations in panic disorder patients and raise the question whether this is also found after long-term exercise training and if it is related to the therapeutic outcome.

[55] Xiong, G. L., et al.   Does meditation enhance cognition and brain plasticity?   Ann N Y Acad Sci. 1172:63-69, 2009.   Department of Psychiatry and Behavioral Sciences, University of California, Davis, Sacramento, California, USA.

Meditation practices have various health benefits including the possibility of preserving cognition and preventing dementia.   While the mechanisms remain investigational, studies show that meditation may affect multiple pathways that could play a role in brain aging and mental fitness.   For example, meditation may reduce stress-induced cortisol secretion and this could have neuroprotective effects potentially via elevating levels of brain derived neurotrophic factor (BDNF).

[56] Neurogenesis in the subventricular zone following transcranial magnetic field stimulation and nigrostriatal lesions.

http://onlinelibrary.wiley.com/doi/10.1111/j.1440-1819.2010.02170.x/full

http://www.molecularbrain.com/content/7/1/11

[57] Fan Y, Liu Z, Weinstein PR, Fike JR, Liu J (January 2007). "Environmental enrichment enhances neurogenesis and improves functional outcome after cranial irradiation". Eur. J. Neurosci. 25 (1): 38–46. doi:10.1111/j.1460-9568.2006.05269.x. PMID 17241265.

Veena J, Srikumar BN, Mahati K, Bhagya V, Raju TR, Shankaranarayana Rao BS (March 2009). "Enriched environment restores hippocampal cell proliferation and ameliorates cognitive deficits in chronically stressed rats". J. Neurosci. Res. 87 (4): 831–43. doi:10.1002/jnr.21907. PMID 19006089.

Meshi D, Drew MR, Saxe M, et al. (June 2006). "Hippocampal neurogenesis is not required for behavioral effects of environmental enrichment". Nat. Neurosci. 9 (6): 729–31. doi:10.1038/nn1696. PMID 16648847.

Rampon C, Jiang CH, Dong H, et al. (November 2000). "Effects of environmental enrichment on gene expression in the brain". *Proc. Natl. Acad. Sci. U.S.A.* **97** (23): 12880–4. doi:10.1073/pnas.97.23.12880. PMC 18858. PMID 11070096.

Ickes BR, Pham TM, Sanders LA, Albeck DS, Mohammed AH, Granholm AC (July 2000). "Long-term environmental enrichment leads to regional increases in neurotrophin levels in rat brain". *Exp. Neurol.* **164** (1): 45–52. doi:10.1006/exnr.2000.7415. PMID 10877914.

http://www.kaganonline.com/free_articles/dr_spencer_kagan/287/Raising-Smarter-Children-Creating-an-Enriched-Learning-Environment

[58] Serum BDNF Concentrations Show Strong Seasonal Variation and Correlations with the Amount of Ambient Sunlight

[59] Impact of age and caloric restriction on neurogenesis in the dentate gyrus of C57BL/6 mice.

[60] Calorie restriction alleviates the age-related decrease in neural progenitor cell division in the aging brain.

[61] http://www.ncbi.nlm.nih.gov/pubmed/18201870

http://www.researchgate.net/publication/51403574_Ketogenic_diet_does_not_disturb_neurogenesis_in_the_dentate_gyrus_in_rats

[62] Sexual Experience Promotes Adult Neurogenesis in the Hippocampus Despite an Initial Elevation in Stress Hormones

[63] Sleep and Adult Neurogenesis: Implications for Cognition and Mood.

http://www.sciencedirect.com/science/article/pii/S0361923006000426

Sleep deprivation inhibits adult neurogenesis in the hippocampus by elevating glucocorticoids

[64]

http://www.sciencemag.org/content/335/6073/1175.summary?sid=aa2c4fc0-e46a-4b58-bf4f-7dd56ffbf4f5

Activation of adult-born neurons facilitates learning and memory.

[65] Taglialatela, G., et al. Stimulation of nerve growth factor receptors in PC12 by acetyl-L-carnitine. Biochem Pharmacol. 44(3):577-85, 1992.

Department of Human Biological Chemistry and Genetics, University of Texas Medical Branch, Galveston, USA.

Acetyl-L-carnitine (Acetyl-L-Carnitine (ALCAR)) prevents some deficits associated with aging in the central nervous system (CNS), such as the aged-related reduction of nerve growth factor (NGF) binding. The aim of this study was to ascertain whether Acetyl-L-Carnitine (ALCAR) could affect the expression of an NGF receptor (p75NGFR). Treatment of PC12 cells with Acetyl-L-Carnitine (ALCAR) increased equilibrium binding of 125I-NGF. Acetyl-L-Carnitine (ALCAR) treatment also increased the amount of immunoprecipitable p75NGFR from PC12 cells. Lastly, the level of p75NGFR messenger RNA (mRNA) in PC12 was increased following Acetyl-L-Carnitine (ALCAR) treatment. These results are in agreement with the hypothesis that there is a direct action of Acetyl-L-Carnitine (ALCAR) on p75NGFR expression in aged rodent CNS.

[66] Tirassa, P., et al. High-dose anabolic androgenic steroids modulate concentrations of nerve growth factor and expression of its low affinity receptor (p75-NGFr) in male rat brain. Journal of Neuroscience Research. 47:198-207, 1997.

[67] Wrann CD, White JP, Salogiannnis J, Laznik-Bogoslavski D, Wu J, Ma D, Lin JD, Greenberg ME, Spiegelman BM (November 2013). "Exercise Induces Hippocampal BDNF through a PGC-1α/FNDC5 Pathway". *Cell Metab.* 18 (5): 649–59. doi:10.1016/j.cmet.2013.09.008. PMID 24120943.

Fuss J, Biedermann SV, Falfán-Melgoza C, Auer MK, Zheng L, Steinle J, Hörner F, Sartorius A, Ende G, Weber-Fahr W, Gass P (November 2013). "Exercise boosts hippocampal volume by preventing early age-related gray matter loss". *Hippocampus* 24 (2): 131–4. doi:10.1002/hipo.22227. PMID 24178895. Lay summary – *Nature Magazine.*

[68]

http://www.psychologytoday.com/blog/the-athletes-way/201402/irisin-the-exercise-hormone-has-powerful-health-benefits

[69] Vega, J. A., et al.   Nerve growth factor receptor immunoreactivity in the cerebellar cortex of aged rats: effect of choline alfoscerate treatment.   Mech Ageing Dev.   69(1-2):119-27, 1993.

[70] http://www.jneurosci.org/content/8/7/2394

[71] Barry S. R.   Clinical implications of basic neuroscience research. II: NMDA Receptors and neurotrophic factors. [review].   Archives of Physical Medicine & Rehabilitation.   72(13):1095-1101, 1991.

Hefti, F., et al.   Nerve growth factor and Alzheimer's disease. [review].   Clinical Neuropharmacology. 14(Suppl 1):S62-76, 1991.

Knusel, B., et al.   Neurotrophins and Alzheimer's disease: beyond cholinergic neurons.   Life Sciences. 58(22):2019-2027, 1996.

Lapchak, P. A: Nerve growth factor pharmacology: Application to the treatment of cholinergic neurodegeneration in Alzheimer's disease.   Experimental Neurology. 124(1):16-20, 1993.

Olson, L.   NGF and the treatment of Alzheimer's disease.   Experimental Neurology.   124(1):5-15, 1993.

Seiger A, et al.   Intracranial infusion of purified nerve growth factor to an Alzheimer patient: The first attempt of a possible future treatment strategy. Behavioural Brain Research.   57(2):255-61, 1993.

[72] Lukoyanov, N. V., et al.   Nerve growth factor improves spatial learning and restores hippocampal cholinergic fibers in rats withdrawn from chronic treatment with ethanol.   Exp Brain Res.   148(1):88-94, 2003.

[73] Emanuele, E., et al.   Raised plasma nerve growth factor levels associated with early-stage romantic love. Psychoneuroendocrinology.   31(3):288-294, 2006.

[74] Hefti, F., et al.   Nerve growth factor and Alzheimer's disease. [review].   Clinical Neuropharmacology. 14(Suppl 1):S62-S76, 1991.

[75] Hefti, F., et al.   Nerve growth factor and Alzheimer's disease. [review].   Clinical Neuropharmacology. 14(Suppl 1):S62-76, 1991.

[76] Effects of huperzine A on memory deficits and neurotrophic factors production after transient cerebral ischemia and reperfusion in mice

[77] Potentiation of nerve growth factor-induced neurite outgrowth in PC12 cells by a Coptidis Rhizoma extract and protoberberine alkaloids.

http://www.ncbi.nlm.nih.gov/pmc/articles/PMC3308712/

http://www.tandfonline.com/doi/pdf/10.1271/bbb.66.2491

[78] Acetyl-L-carnitine treatment increases nerve growth factor levels and choline acetyltransferase activity in the central nervous system of aged rats.

[79] Nerve growth factor-inducing activity of Hericium erinaceus in 1321N1 human astrocytoma cells.

[80] Bioactive Substances in YAMABUSHITAKE, the Hericium erinaceum, Fungus, and its Medicinal Utilization, Takashi Mizuno, Shizuoka University

Kolotushkina, E. V.; Moldavan, M. G.; Voronin, K. Y.; Skibo, G. G. (2003). "The influence of Hericium erinaceus extract on myelination process in vitro". *Fiziolohichnyi zhurnal* 49 (1): 38–45

Kawagishi, H., et al. Erinacines A, B, and C, strong stimulators of nerve growth factor synthesis, from the mycelia of Hericium erinaceum. Tetrahedron Lett. 35: 1569-1572, 1994

Kawagishi, H., et al. Erinacine D, a stimulator of NGF-synthesis, from the mycelia of Hericium erinaceum. Heterocycl Commun. 2: 51-54, 1996

Kawagishi, H. The inducer of the synthesis of nerve growth factor from lion's mane (Hericium erinaceus). Explore. 11(4), 2002

Nerve growth factor-inducing activity of Hericium erinaceus in 1321N1 human astrocytoma cells

The influence of Hericium erinaceus extract on myelination process in vitro

Improving effects of the mushroom Yamabushitake (Hericium erinaceus) on mild cognitive impairment: a double-blind placebo-controlled clinical trial

Effect of an exo-polysaccharide from the culture broth of Hericium erinaceus on enhancement of growth and differentiation of rat adrenal nerve cells

[81] Effect of Astragalus membranaceus in rats on peripheral nerve regeneration: in vitro and in vivo studies.

[82] Soumyanath A, *et al.* Centella asiatica accelerates nerve regeneration upon oral administration and contains multiple active fractions increasing neurite elongation in-vitro. *J Pharm Pharmacol.* (2005)

[83] *Codonopsis pilosula* (Franch) Nannf total alkaloids potentiate neurite outgrowth induced by nerve growth factor in PC12 cells

[84] Cistanches Herba enhances learning and memory by inducing nerve growth factor

[85] Isorhamnetin, A Flavonol Aglycone from Ginkgo biloba L., Induces Neuronal Differentiation of Cultured PC12 Cells: Potentiating the Effect of Nerve Growth Factor.

[86] Yabe T., Tuchida H., Kiyohara H., Takeda T., Yamada H. (2003). "Induction of NGF synthesis in astrocytes by onjisaponins of *Polygala tenuifolia*, constituents of kampo (Japanese herbal) medicine, Ninjin-yoei-to.". *Phytomedicine* 10 (2-3): 106–14. doi:10.1078/094471103321659799. PMID 12725562

Yabe T1, *et al.* Enhancements of choline acetyltransferase activity and nerve growth factor secretion by Polygalae radix-extract containing active ingredients in Kami-untan-to. *Phytomedicine.* (1997)

[87] Carnosic Acid, a Component of Rosemary (*Rosmarinus officinalis* L.), Promotes Synthesis of Nerve Growth Factor in T98G Human Glioblastoma Cells

[88] Takara's Scientists Discover Compounds Enhancing in Vivo Production of Nerve Growth Factor

[89] Effects of American ginseng (*Panax quinquefolius*) on neurocognitive function: an acute, randomised, double-blind, placebo-controlled, crossover study   Andrew Scholey, Anastasia Ossoukhova, [...], and Con Stough

[90] [Effect of radix Rehmanniae preparata on the expression of c-fos and NGF in hippocampi and learning and memory in rats with damaged thalamic arcuate nucleus].

[91] Shigeta K, *et al*. Potentiation of nerve growth factor-induced neurite outgrowth in PC12 cells by a Coptidis Rhizoma extract and protoberberine alkaloids. *Biosci Biotechnol Biochem*. (2002)

Lee MK, Kim HS. Inhibitory effects of protoberberine alkaloids from the roots of Coptis japonica on catecholamine biosynthesis in PC12 cells. *Planta Med*. (1996)Hsieh MT, *et al*. Effects of palmatine on motor activity and the concentration of central monoamines and its metabolites in rats. *Jpn J Pharmacol*. (1993)

Shin JS, *et al*. Inhibition of dopamine biosynthesis by protoberberine alkaloids in PC12 cells. *Neurochem Res*. (2000)

[92] Hamada N, *et al*. Metabolites of sesamin, a major lignan in sesame seeds, induce neuronal differentiation in PC12 cells through activation of ERK1/2 signaling pathway. *J Neural Transm*. (2009)

[93] Dubal, D. B., et al.   Estradiol: a protective and trophic factor in the brain.   Alzheimer's Disease Review. 4:1-9, 1999.

Several studies suggest that estradiol may exert growth promoting effects by influencing the expression of nerve growth factor.

Gibbs, R. B.   Estrogen and nerve growth factor related systems in the brain.   Annals of the New York Academy of Sciences, USA.   743:165-196, 1994.

Miranda, R. C., et al.   Presumptive estrogen target neurons express mRNAs for both the neurotrophins and neurotrophin receptors: a basis for potential developmental interactions of estrogen with the neurotrophins. Mol Cell Neurosci.   4:510-525, 1993.

[94] Tirassa, P., et al.   High-dose anabolic androgenic steroids modulate concentrations of nerve growth factor and expression of its low affinity receptor (p75-NGFr) in male rat brain.   Journal of Neuroscience Research. 47:198-207, 1997.

[95] http://www.neurobiologyofaging.org/article/S0197-4580(04)00163-0/abstract

[96] Melatonin increases nerve growth factor in mouse submandibular gland.

[97] Membrane fatty acid modifications of PC12 cells by arachidonate or docosahexaenoate affect neurite outgrowth but not norepinephrine release.

[98] Nunzi, M. G., et al.   Therapeutic properties of phosphatidylserine in the aging brain.   In: Hanin, I., Pepeu, G., editors.   Phospholipids: Biochemical, Pharmacological, and Analytical Considerations.   New York: Plenum Press;   1990.

[99] Noopept stimulates the expression of NGF and BDNF in rat hippocampus.

[100] Mizuta, I., et al.   Selegiline and desmethylselegiline stimulate NGF, BDNF, and GDNF synthesis in cultured mouse astrocytes.   Biochem Biophys Res Commun.   279(3):751-755, 2000.

[101] Dean, W. & Morgenthaler, J. Smart Drugs & Nutrients. B & J Publications, Santa Cruz, California, USA. 1990:118.

[102] Mason, R. Idebenone, a drug with a myriad of antiaging benefits. Anti-Aging Bulletin. 4(4):22-25, 1999.

[103] Nishio, T., et al. Repeated injections of nicergoline increase the nerve growth factor level in the aged rat brain. Jpn J Pharmacol. 76(3):321-3, 1998.

[104] http://www.ncbi.nlm.nih.gov/pmc/articles/PMC1852434/

[105] Neary JT, et al. Trophic actions of extracellular nucleotides and nucleosides on glial and neuronal cells. Trends Neurosci. (1996)

Boglári G, Szeberényi J. Nerve growth factor in combination with second messenger analogues causes neuronal differentiation of PC12 cells expressing a dominant inhibitory Ras protein without inducing activation of extracellular signal-regulated kinases. Eur J Neurosci. (2001)

Chuang HH, et al. Bradykinin and nerve growth factor release the capsaicin receptor from PtdIns(4,5)P2-mediated inhibition. Nature. (2001)

Rathbone MP, et al. Trophic effects of purines in neurons and glial cells. Prog Neurobiol. (1999)

Wang L, et al. Dietary uridine-5'-monophosphate supplementation increases potassium-evoked dopamine release and promotes neurite outgrowth in aged rats. J Mol Neurosci. (2005)

[106] http://www.ncbi.nlm.nih.gov/pubmed/21379380

http://www.ncbi.nlm.nih.gov/pubmed/11722606

http://www.ncbi.nlm.nih.gov/pubmed/11418861

http://www.ncbi.nlm.nih.gov/pubmed/16365320

http://www.ncbi.nlm.nih.gov/pubmed/22528682

[107] Quercetin stimulates NGF-induced neurite outgrowth in PC12 cells via activation of Na(+)/K(+)/2Cl(-) cotransporter.

[108] · Shinoda, I., et al. Lactoferrin promotes nerve growth factor synthesis/secretion in mouse fibroblast L-M cells. Advances in Experimental Medicine and Biology. 357:279-385, 1994.

[109] Physiological Importance of Quinoenzymes and the O-Quinone Family of Cofactors

[110] Turmeric compound boosts regeneration of brain stem cells

[111] High-dose dietary supplementation of vitamin A induces brain-derived neurotrophic factor and nerve growth factor production in mice with simultaneous deficiency of vitamin A and zinc.

[112] Kiraly, S. J., et al. Vitamin D as a neuroactive substance: review. Scientific World Journal. 6:125-139, 2006.

McGrath, J. J., et al. Vitamin D(3)-implications for brain development. J Steroid Biochem Mol Biol. 89-90:557-560, 2004.

Neveu, I., et al. 1,25-dihydroxyvitamin D3 regulates the synthesis of nerve growth factor in primary cultures of glial cells. Brain Research. Molecular Brain Research. 24(1-4):70-76, 1994.

Saporito, M. S., et al.   Pharmacological induction of nerve growth factor mRNA in adult rat brain.   Exp Neurol.   123(2):295-302, 1993.

[113] Pandey, S. C., et al.   Effector immediate-early gene arc in the amygdala plays a critical role in alcoholism.   Journal of Neuroscience.   28(10):2589-2600, 2008.

[114] Strohle, A., et al.   Acute exercise ameliorates reduced brain-derived neurotrophic factor in patients with panic disorder.   Psychoneuroendocrinology.   2009.

Kobayashi, K., et al.   Serum brain-derived neurotrophic factor (BDNF) levels in patients with panic disorder: as a biological predictor of response to group cognitive behavioral therapy.   Prog Neuropsychopharmacol Biol Psychiatry.   29(5):658-663, 2005.

[115] Lebrun, B., et al.   Brain-derived neurotrophic factor (BDNF) and food intake regulation: a minireview.   Auton Neurosci.   126-127:30-38, 2006.

Pelleymounter, M. A., et al.   Characteristics of BDNF-induced weight loss.   Exp Neurol.   131(2):229-238, 1995.

Stanek, K., et al.   Serum brain-derived neurotrophic factor is associated with reduced appetite in healthy older adults.   J Nutr Health Aging.   12(3):183-185, 2008.

[116] Knusel, B., et al.   Neurotrophins and Alzheimer's disease: beyond the cholinergic neurons.   Life Sciences.   58(22):2019-2027, 1996.

Liu, Z., et al.   [The research advance of brain derived neurotrophic factor.]   Sheng Wu Yi Xue Gong Cheng Xue Za Zhi.   17(4):454-446, 2000.

[117] Dwivedi, Y.   Brain-derived neurotrophic factor: role in depression and suicide.   Neuropsychiatr Dis Treat.   5:433-449, 2009.

[118] Bekinschtein, P., et al.   BDNF is essential to promote persistence of long-term memory storage.   Proc Natl Acad Sci U S A. 105(7): 2711–2716,   2008.

[119] A simple role for BDNF in learning and memory?

Role for brain-derived neurotrophic factor in learning and memory.

Microglia Promote Learning-Dependent Synapse Formation through Brain-Derived Neurotrophic Factor

[120] http://www.jneurosci.org/content/20/18/7116.full.pdf

Involvement of BDNF receptor TrkB in spatial memory formation.

[121] Cholinergic regulation of brain-derived neurotrophic factor (BDNF) and nerve growth factor (NGF) but not neurotrophin-3 (NT-3) mRNA levels in the developing rat hippocampus.

BDNF is a neurotrophic factor for dopaminergic neurons of the substantia nigra.

http://www.jneurosci.org/content/22/17/7580.full.pdf

[122] Serum levels of brain-derived neurotrophic factor correlate with motor impairment in Parkinson's disease.

[123] Chen, D. C., et al.   Decreased levels of serum brain-derived neurotrophic factor in drug-naïve first-episode schizophrenia: relationship to clinical phenotypes.   Psychopharmacology (Berl).   2009.

[124] Evidence that brain-derived neurotrophic factor is a trophic factor for motor neurons in vivo.

[125] Wang,.Z. F., et al. Effects of huperzine A on memory deficits and neurotrophic factors production after transient cerebral ischemia and reperfusion in mice. Pharmacol Biochem Behav. 83(4):603-611, 2006.

[126]

http://www.ncnp.go.jp/nin/guide/r3/staff/numakawa_files/Journal%20of%20Biological%20Medicine%20%20Numakawa.pdf

http://www.ncbi.nlm.nih.gov/pubmed/21617527

[127] http://www.ergo-log.com/betaalanineanxiety.html

[128] The memory-enhancing effects of Euphoria longan fruit extract in mice.

[129] Williams, C. M., et al. Blueberry-induced changes in spatial working memory correlate with changes in hippocampal CREB phosphorylation and brain-derived neurotrophic factor (BDNF) levels. Free Radic Biol Med. 2008.

[130] http://www.sciencedaily.com/releases/2013/04/130412132229.htm

[131] Labelle C, Leclerc N. Exogenous BDNF, NT-3 and NT-4 differentially regulate neurite outgrowth in cultured hippocampal neurons. Brain Res Dev Brain Res. (2000)

[132] Li, Q., et al. Long-term administration of green tea catechins prevents age-related spatial learning and memory decline in C57BL/6 J mice by regulating hippocampal cyclic amp-response element binding protein signaling cascade. Neuroscience. 159(4):1208-1215, 2009.

[133] Zhao, H., et al Long-term ginsenoside administration prevents memory impairment in aged C57BL/6J mice by up-regulating the synaptic plasticity-related proteins in hippocampus. Behav Brain Res. 201(2):311-317, 2009.

[134] Wang, Z., et al. Catalpol ameliorates beta amyloid-induced degeneration of cholinergic neurons by elevating brain-derived neurotrophic factors. Neuroscience. 2009.

[135] Hong SW, et al. Gypenoside TN-2 ameliorates scopolamine-induced learning deficit in mice. J Ethnopharmacol. (2011)

http://www.ijrpbsonline.com/files/RV12.pdf

[136] http://www.ncbi.nlm.nih.gov/pubmed/25004888

[137]

http://emoryott.technologypublisher.com/tech/Gedunin_and_its_Derivatives_Useful_for_Treatment_of_Neurodegenerative_Diseases

[138] Melatonin Precursor Stimulates Growth Factor Circuits in Brain

[139] Dubal, D. B., et al. Estradiol: a protective and trophic factor in the brain. Alzheimer's Disease Review. 4:1-9, 1999.

Singh, M. The effect of overiectomy and estradiol replacement on brain-derived neurotrophic factor messenger ribonucleic acid expression in cortical and hippocampal brain regions of female Sprague-Dawley rats. Endocrinology. 136(5):2320-2324, 1995.

[140] De Nicola, A. F., et al. Progesterone treatment of spinal cord injury: effects on receptors, neurotrophins, and myelination. J Mol Neurosci. 28(1):3-15, 2006.

Gonzalez, S. L., et al. Progesterone up-regulates neuronal brain-derived neurotrophic factor expression in the injured spinal cord. Neuroscience. 125(3):605-614, 2004.

Gonzalez, S. L., et al. Progesterone neuroprotection in spinal cord trauma involves up-regulation of brain-derived neurotrophic factor in motoneurons. J Steroid Biochem Mol Biol. 94(1-3):143-149, 2005.

Gonzalez, Progesterone modulates brain-derived neurotrophic factor and choline acetyltransferase in degenerating Wobbler motoneurons. Exp Neurol. 203(2):406-414, 2007.

[141] Cole, G. M., et al. Docosahexaenoic acid (DHA) may prevent age-related dementia. Journal of Nutrition. 2010.

Jiang, L. H., et al. The influence of orally administered docosahexaenoic acid on cognitive ability in aged mice. J Nutr Biochem. 2008.

Levant, B., et al. Decreased brain docosahexaenoic acid content produces neurobiological effects associated with depression: interactions with reproductive status in female rats. Psychoneuroendocrinology. 2008.

[142] Bousquet, M., et al. Modulation of brain-derived neurotrophic factor as a potential neuroprotective mechanism of action of omega-3 in a parkinsonian animal model. Prog Neuropsychopharmacol Biol Psychiatry. 2009.

[143] Royal Jelly and Its Unique Fatty Acid, 10-Hydroxy-Trans-2-Decenoic Acid, Promote Neurogenesis by Neural Stem/progenitor Cells in Vitro. Biomedical Research (Tokyo, Japan) 28(5): 261–266.

H. Ito, A. Nakajima, H. Nomoto, and S. Furukawa, "Neurotrophins facilitate neuronal differentiation of cultured neural stem cells via induction of mRNA expression of basic helix-loop-helix transcription factors Mash1 and Math1," Journal of Neuroscience Res

[144] http://www.ncbi.nlm.nih.gov/pubmed/22016520

[145] Kling, M. A., et al. Rat brain and serum lithium concentrations after acute injections of lithium carbonate and orotate. J Pharm Pharmacol. 30(6):368-370, 1978

The clinical application of lithium orotate Nieper, H.A.. Agressologie. 14(6):407-411, 1973

Fugate, L. Potential role for lithium in preventing Alzheimer's disease. Vitamin Research News. 16(2), 2002

Hashimoto, R., et al. [Neuroprotective actions of lithium.] Seishin Shinkeigaku Zasshi. 105(1):81-86, 2003

Hashimoto, R., et al. Lithium induces brain-derived neurotrophic factor and activates TrkB in rodent cortical neurons: an essential step for neuroprotection against glutamate excitotoxicity. Neuropharmacology. 43(7):1173-1179, 2002

[146] Nowak, G., et al. Zinc treatment induces cortical brain-derived neurotrophic factor gene expression. Eur J Pharmacol. 492(1):57-59, 2004.

Sowa-Kucma, M., et al. Antidepressant-like activity of zinc: further behavioral and molecular evidence. J Neural Transm. 2008.

[147] Dolotov OV, Karpenko EA, Inozemtseva LS, Seredenina TS, Levitskaya NG, Rozyczka J, Dubynina EV, Novosadova EV, Andreeva LA, Alfeeva LY, Kamensky AA, Grivennikov IA, Myasoedov NF, Engele J (October 2006). "Semax, an analog of ACTH(4-10) with cognitive effects, regulates BDNF and trkB expression in the rat hippocampus". Brain Res. 1117 (1): 54–60. doi:10.1016/j.brainres.2006.07.108. PMID 16996037

[148] http://www.scirp.org/journal/PaperInformation.aspx?PaperID=40560#.U9VYWfldVWg

http://www.sciencedirect.com/science/article/pii/S0006899306022955

http://link.springer.com/article/10.1023%2FA%3A1025177812262

[149] Noopept stimulates the expression of NGF and BDNF in rat hippocampus (Bull Exp Biol Med. 2008 Sep;146(3):334-7).

[150] Mizuta, I., et al. Selegiline and desmethylselegiline stimulate NGF, BDNF, and GDNF synthesis in cultured mouse astrocytes. Biochem Biophys Res Commun. 279(3):751-755, 2000.

[151] Pearson, D., et al. Enriched environment may reduce apoptosis in the brain. The Durk Pearson & Sandy Shaw Life Extension News. 2(4), 1999.

[152] Giardino, L., et al. Neuroprotection and aging of the cholinergic system: a role for the ergoline derivative nicergoline (Sermion). Neuroscience. 109(3):487-497, 2002.

Mizuno, T., et al. Protective effects of nicergoline against neuronal cell death induced by activated microglia and astrocytes. Brain Research. 1066(1-2):78-85, 2005.

[153] Jang SW1, et al. A selective TrkB agonist with potent neurotrophic activities by 7,8-dihydroxyflavone. Proc Natl Acad Sci U S A. (2010)

Liu X1, et al. A synthetic 7,8-dihydroxyflavone derivative promotes neurogenesis and exhibits potent antidepressant effect. J Med Chem. (2010)

[154] http://www.pnas.org/content/107/6/2687.long

Liu X, Obianyo O, Chan CB, Huang J, Xue S, Yang JJ et al. (2014). "Biochemical and biophysical investigation of the brain-derived neurotrophic factor mimetic 7,8-dihydroxyflavone in the binding and activation of the TrkB receptor". J. Biol. Chem. 289 (40): 27571–84. doi:10.1074/jbc.M114.562561. PMID 25143381.

Zeng Y, Wang X, Wang Q, Liu S, Hu X, McClintock SM (2013). "Small molecules activating TrkB receptor for treating a variety of CNS disorders". CNS Neurol Disord Drug Targets 12 (7): 1066–77. PMID 23844685

[155] http://www.ncbi.nlm.nih.gov/pmc/articles/PMC3150605/

[156] Wang, R., et al. Curcumin protects against glutamate excitotoxicity in rat cerebral cortical neurons by increasing brain-derived neurotrophic factor level and activating TrkB. Brain Res. 2008.

Xu, Y., et al. Curcumin reverses the effects of chronic stress on behavior, the HPA axis, BDNF expression and phosphorylation of CREB. Brain Research. 1122(1):56-64, 2006.

Xu, Y., et al. Curcumin reverses impaired hippocampal neurogenesis and increases serotonin receptor 1A mRNA and brain-derived neurotrophic factor expression in chronically stressed rats. Brain Research. 2007.

[157] Quercetin attenuates cell apoptosis in focal cerebral ischemia rat brain via activation of BDNF-TrkB-PI3K/Akt signaling pathway.

[158] Jana A, Modi KK, Roy A, Anderson JA, van Breemen RB, Pahan K. Up-regulation of neurotrophic factors by cinnamon and its metabolite sodium benzoate: therapeutic implications for neurodegenerative disorders. J Neuroimmune Pharmacol. 2013 Mar 9

[159] Kheirvari, S., et al.   High-dose dietary supplementation of vitamin A induces brain-derived neurotrophic factor and nerve growth factor production in mice with simultaneous deficiency of vitamin A and zinc.   Nutr Neurosci.   11(5):228-234, 2008.

[160] Tsai, S. J.   Cysteamine-related agents could be potential antidepressants through increasing central BDNF levels.   Med Hypotheses.   67(5):1185-1188, 2006.

[161] Airaksinen M, Saarma M (2002). "The GDNF family: signalling, biological functions and therapeutic value". Nat Rev Neurosci 3 (5): 383–94. doi:10.1038/nrn812. PMID 11988777

[162] http://www.researchgate.net/publication/258059282_Doxycycline-regulated_GDNF_expression_promotes_axonal_regeneration_and_functional_recovery_in_transected_peripheral_nerve

[163] GDNF promotes neurite outgrowth and upregulates galectin-1 through the RET/PI3K signaling in cultured adult rat dorsal root ganglion neurons.

[164] Jankovic, J.   New and emerging therapies for Parkinson disease.   Arch Neurol.   56:785-790, 1990.

One particularly promising therapeutic and potentially neuroprotective approach to the treatment of Parkinson's disease involves the use of neurotrophic factors, particularly glial cell line-derived neurotrophic factor (GDNF).

Lapchak, P. A.   A preclinical development strategy designed to optimize the use of glial cell-line derived neurotrophic factor in the treatment of Parkinson's disease.   Mov Disord.   13(Supplement 1):49-54, 1998.

GDNF is reported to enhance the survival of midbrain dopaminergic neurons in vitro and to rescue degenerating neurons in vivo.

Miyoshi, Y., et al.   Glial cell line-derived neurotrophic factor-levodopa interaction and reduction of side effects in parkinsonian monkeys.   Ann Neurol.   42:208-214, 1997.

Intraventricular administration of GDNF in experimental monkeys ameliorates parkinsonian findings, reduces the adverse effects of L-dopa and results in a 20% enlargement of nigral neurons accompanied by increased fiber density.

[165] Jankovic, J.   New and emerging therapies for Parkinson disease.   Arch Neurol.   56:785-790, 1990.

One particularly promising therapeutic and potentially neuroprotective approach to the treatment of Parkinson's disease involves the use of neurotrophic factors, particularly glial cell line-derived neurotrophic factor (GDNF).

Lapchak, P. A.   A preclinical development strategy designed to optimize the use of glial cell-line derived neurotrophic factor in the treatment of Parkinson's disease.   Mov Disord.   13(Supplement 1):49-54, 1998.

GDNF is reported to enhance the survival of midbrain dopaminergic neurons in vitro and to rescue degenerating neurons in vivo.

Miyoshi, Y., et al.   Glial cell line-derived neurotrophic factor-levodopa interaction and reduction of side effects in parkinsonian monkeys.   Ann Neurol.   42:208-214, 1997.

Intraventricular administration of GDNF in experimental monkeys ameliorates parkinsonian findings, reduces the adverse effects of L-dopa and results in a 20% enlargement of nigral neurons accompanied by increased fiber density.

[166] Zheng, S. X., et al.   Bilobalide promotes expression of glial cell line-derived neurotrophic factor and vascular endothelial growth factor in rat astrocytes.   Acta Pharmacol Sin.   21(2):151-155, 2000.

[167] Rehmannia glutinosa induces glial cell line-derived neurotrophic factor gene expression in astroglial cells via cPKC and ERK1/2 pathways independently

[168] http://www.ncbi.nlm.nih.gov/pmc/articles/PMC2765306/

[169] Armstrong, K. J., et al.   Induction of GDNF mRNA expression by melatonin in rat C6 glioma cells.   Neuroreport.   13(4):473-475, 2002.

Chen, K. B., et al.   Oxidative injury to the locus coeruleus of rat brain: neuroprotection by melatonin.   J Pineal Res.   35(2):109-117, 2003.

Tang, Y. P., et al.   Enhanced glial cell line-derived neurotrophic factor mRNA expression upon (-)-deprenyl and melatonin treatments.   J Neurosci Res.   53(5):593-604, 1998.

[170] Hashimoto, M., et al.   Oral administration of royal jelly facilitates mRNA expression of glial cell line-derived neurotrophic factor and neurofilament h in the hippocampus of the adult mouse brain.   Biosci Biotechnol Biochem.   69(4):800-805, 2005.

[171] Mizuta, I., et al.   Selegiline and desmethylselegiline stimulate NGF, BDNF, and GDNF synthesis in cultured mouse astrocytes.   Biochem Biophys Res Commun.   279(3):751-755, 2000.

Tang, Y. P., et al.   Enhanced glial cell line-derived neurotrophic factor mRNA expression upon (-)-deprenyl and melatonin treatments.   J Neurosci Res.   53(5):593-604, 1998.

[172] Wang, J. Y., et al.   Vitamin D(3) attenuates 6-hydroxydopamine-induced neurotoxicity in rats.   Brain Research.   904(1):67-75, 2001.

Recent studies have shown that 1,25-dihydroxyvitamin D(3) (calcitriol) enhances endogenous GDNF expression in vitro and in vivo.

[173] Enzinger C, Fazekas F, Matthews PM, et al. Risk factors for progression of brain atrophy in aging: six-year follow-up of normal subjects. Neurology. 2005 May 24;64(10):1704-11.

Hedman AM. Human brain changes across the life span: a review of 56 longitudinal magnetic resonance imaging studies. Human Brain Mapping.   2012;33:1987-220.

[174] Hedman AM. Human brain changes across the life span: a review of 56 longitudinal magnetic resonance imaging studies. Human Brain Mapping.   2012;33:1987-220.

Olesen PJ, Guo X, Gustafson D, et al. A population-based study on the influence of brain atrophy on 20-year survival after age 85. Neurology. 2011 Mar 8;76(10):879-86.

Guo X, Steen B, Matousek M, et al. A population-based study on brain atrophy and motor performance in elderly women. J Gerontol A Biol Sci Med Sci. 2001 Oct;56(10):M633-7.

Henneman WJ, Sluimer JD, Cordonnier C, et al. MRI biomarkers of vascular damage and atrophy predicting mortality in a memory clinic population. Stroke. 2009 Feb;40(2):492-8.

Johansson L, Skoog I, Gustafson DR, et al. Midlife psychological distress associated with late-life brain atrophy and white matter lesions: a 32-year population study of women. Psychosom Med. 2012 Feb-Mar;74(2):120-5.

Olesen PJ, Gustafson DR, Simoni M, et al. Temporal lobe atrophy and white matter lesions are related to major depression over 5 years in the elderly. Neuropsychopharmacology. 2010 Dec;35(13):2638-45.

[175] Fjell A et al. Structural brain changes in aging: courses, causes and cognitive consequences. Revs Neurosci. 2010; 21(3):182-221.

Fjell A et al. Structural brain changes in aging: courses, causes and cognitive consequences. Revs Neurosci. 2010; 21(3):182-221.

Fjell A et al. Structural brain changes in aging: courses, causes and cognitive consequences. Revs Neurosci. 2010; 21(3):182-221.

[176] Draganski B, Lutti A, Kherif F. Impact of brain aging and neurodegeneration on cognition: evidence from MRI. Curr Opin Neurol. 2013 Dec;26(6):640-5.

[177] Homocysteine-Lowering by B Vitamins Slows the Rate of Accelerated Brain Atrophy in Mild Cognitive Impairment: A Randomized Controlled Trial

[178] Poor sleep quality is associated with increased cortical atrophy in community-dwelling adults

[179] Blood Pressure and Progression of Brain AtrophyThe SMART-MR Study

Alosco ML, Brickman AM, Spitznagel MB, et al. Independent and interactive effects of blood pressure and cardiac function on brain volume and white matter hyperintensities in heart failure. J Am Soc Hypertens. 2013 Sep-Oct;7(5):336-43.

Iadecola C, Davisson RL. Hypertension and cerebrovascular dysfunction. Cell Metab. 2008 Jun;7(6):476-84.

Jennings JR, Mendelson DN, Muldoon MF, et al. Regional grey matter shrinks in hypertensive individuals despite successful lowering of blood pressure. J Hum Hypertens. 2012 May;26(5):295-305.

[180] Liu Y, Zhu X, Feinberg D, et al. Arterial spin labeling MRI study of age and gender effects on brain perfusion hemodynamics. Magn Reson Med. 2012 Sep;68(3):912-22.

[181] Brain atrophy linked with cognitive decline in diabetes

[182] Kiliaan AJ, Arnoldussen IA, Gustafson DR. Adipokines: a link between obesity and dementia? Lancet Neurol. 2014 Sep;13(9):913-23.

Raji CA, Ho AJ, Parikshak NN, et al. Brain structure and obesity. Hum Brain Mapp. 2010 Mar;31(3):353-64.

[183] Kubota K, Matsuzawa T, Fujiwara T, et al. Age-related brain atrophy enhanced by smoking: a quantitative study with computed tomography. Tohoku J Exp Med. 1987 Dec;153(4):303-11.

Durazzo TC, Meyerhoff DJ, Nixon SJ. Chronic cigarette smoking: implications for neurocognition and brain neurobiology. Int J Environ Res Public Health. 2010 Oct;7(10):3760-91.

Durazzo TC, Insel PS, Weiner MW. Greater regional brain atrophy rate in healthy elderly subjects with a history of cigarette smoking. Alzheimers Dement. 2012 Nov;8(6):513-9.

[184] Gu Y, Scarmeas N, Short EE, et al. Alcohol intake and brain structure in a multiethnic elderly cohort. Clin Nutr. 2014 Aug;33(4):662-7.

Kubota M, Nakazaki S, Hirai S, Saeki N, Yamaura A, Kusaka T. Alcohol consumption and frontal lobe shrinkage: study of 1432 nonalcoholic subjects. J Neurol Neurosurg Psychiatry. 2001 Jul;71(1):104-6.

Mukamal KJ, Longstreth WT, Jr., Mittleman MA, Crum RM, Siscovick DS. Alcohol consumption and subclinical findings on magnetic resonance imaging of the brain in older adults: the cardiovascular health study. Stroke. 2001 Sep;32(9):1939-46.

[185] Hartman RE, Shah A, Fagan AM, et al. Pomegranate juice decreases amyloid load and improves behavior in a mouse model of Alzheimer's disease. Neurobiol Dis. 2006 Dec;24(3):506-15.

Kumar S, Maheshwari KK, Singh V. Protective effects of Punica granatum seeds extract against aging and scopolamine induced cognitive impairments in mice. Afr J Tradit Complement Altern Med. 2008;6(1):49-56.

Rojanathammanee L, Puig KL, Combs CK. Pomegranate polyphenols and extract inhibit nuclear factor of activated T-cell activity and microglial activation in vitro and in a transgenic mouse model of Alzheimer disease. J Nutr. 2013 May;143(5):597-605.

Choi SJ, Lee JH, Heo HJ, et al. Punica granatum protects against oxidative stress in PC12 cells and oxidative stress-induced Alzheimer's symptoms in mice. J Med Food. 2011 Jul-Aug;14(7-8):695-701.

Bookheimer SY, Renner BA, Ekstrom A, et al. Pomegranate juice augments memory and FMRI activity in middle-aged and older adults with mild memory complaints. Evid Based Complement Alternat Med. 2013;2013:946298.

[186] Hennebelle M, Champeil-Potokar G, Lavialle M, Vancassel S, Denis I. Omega-3 polyunsaturated fatty acids and chronic stress-induced modulations of glutamatergic neurotransmission in the hippocampus. Nutr Rev. 2014 Feb;72(2):99-112.

Tatebayashi Y, Nihonmatsu-Kikuchi N, Hayashi Y, Yu X, Soma M, Ikeda K. Abnormal fatty acid composition in the frontopolar cortex of patients with affective disorders. Transl Psychiatry. 2012;2:e204.

Virtanen JK, Siscovick DS, Lemaitre RN, et al. Circulating omega-3 polyunsaturated fatty acids and subclinical brain abnormalities on MRI in older adults: the Cardiovascular Health Study. J Am Heart Assoc. 2013 Oct;2(5):e000305.

Pottala JV, Yaffe K, Robinson JG, Espeland MA, Wallace R, Harris WS. Higher RBC EPA + Docosahexaenoic acid (DHA) corresponds with larger total brain and hippocampal volumes: WHIMS-MRI study. Neurology. 2014 Feb 4;82(5):435-42.

[187] Association of fish oil supplement use with preservation of brain volume and cognitive function.

[188] Moriya J, Chen R, Yamakawa J, Sasaki K, Ishigaki Y, Takahashi T. Resveratrol improves hippocampal atrophy in chronic fatigue mice by enhancing neurogenesis and inhibiting apoptosis of granular cells. Biol Pharm Bull. 2011;34(3):354-9.

Rege SD, Kumar S, Wilson DN, et al. Resveratrol protects the brain of obese mice from oxidative damage. Oxid Med Cell Longev. 2013;2013:419092.

Chang HC, Tai YT, Cherng YG, et al. Resveratrol attenuates high-fat diet-induced disruption of the blood-brain barrier and protects brain neurons from apoptotic insults. J Agric Food Chem. 2014 Apr 16;62(15):3466-75.

Witte AV, Kerti L, Margulies DS, Floel A. Effects of resveratrol on memory performance, hippocampal functional connectivity, and glucose metabolism in healthy older adults. J Neurosci. 2014 Jun 4;34(23):7862-70.

[189] Smith AD, Smith SM, de Jager CA, Whitbread P, Johnston C, et al. (2010) Homocysteine-lowering by B vitamins slows the rate of accelerated brain atrophy in mild cognitive impairment: a randomized controlled trial. PLoS ONE [online journal]. 2010;5(9):e12244.

Erickson KI, Suever BL, Prakash RS, Colcombe SJ, McAuley E, et al. Greater intake of vitamins B6 and B12 spares gray matter in healthy elderly: A voxel-based morphometry study. Brain Res 2008;1199:20-6.

Jack CR, Jr., Shiung MM, Gunter JL, O'Brien PC, Weigand SD, et al. Comparison of different MRI brain atrophy rate measures with clinical disease progression in AD. Neurology 2004;62:591–600.

Kelland K. B vitamins found to halve aging brain shrinkage. Reuters Health, September 9, 2010.

Institute of Medicine, Food and Nutrition Board. Folate. In: Dietary reference intakes for thiamin, riboflavin, niacin, vitamin B6, folate, vitamin B12, pantothenic acid, biotin, and choline. Washington DC: National Academy Press; 1998, 196-305.

B vitamins slow brain atrophy in people with memory problems

[190] Persistence of neurological damage induced by dietary vitamin B-12 deficiency in infancy.

[191] Kulkarni SK, Dhir A (December 2009). "Berberine: a plant alkaloid with therapeutic potential for central nervous system disorders". *Phytotherapy Research* **24** (3): 317–24. doi:10.1002/ptr.2968. PMID 19998323.

[192] Ved HS, *et al.* Huperzine A, a potential therapeutic agent for dementia, reduces neuronal cell death caused by glutamate. *Neuroreport.* (1997)

Huperzine A regulates amyloid precursor protein processing via protein kinase C and mitogen-activated protein kinase pathways in neuroblastoma SK-N-SH cells over-expressing wild type human amyloid precursor protein 695

[193] http://examine.com/supplements/Beta-Alanine/

[194] http://www.drweil.com/drw/u/ART03059/Acetyl-LCarnitine-ALCAR.html

[195] Huxtable RJ (1992). "Physiological actions of taurine". *Physiol Rev* **72** (1): 101–163. PMID 1731369

[196] Leszek, J; Inglot, AD; Janusz, M; Lisowski, J; Krukowska, K; Georgiades, JA (1999). "Colostrinin: a proline-rich polypeptide (PRP) complex isolated from ovine colostrum for treatment of Alzheimer's disease. A double-blind, placebo-controlled study". *Archivum immunologiae et therapiae experimentalis* **47** (6): 377–85. PMID 10608295.

Kubis, AM; Janusz, M (2008). "Alzheimer's disease: new prospects in therapy and applied experimental models". *Postepy higieny i medycyny doswiadczalnej (Online)* **62**: 372–92. PMID 18688208.

Bilikiewicz, A; Gaus, W (2004). "Colostrinin (a naturally occurring, proline-rich, polypeptide mixture) in the treatment of Alzheimer's disease". *Journal of Alzheimer's disease : JAD* **6** (1): 17–26. PMID 15004324.

[197]
http://www.webmd.com/vitamins-supplements/ingredientmono-1053-theanine.aspx?activeingredientid=1053&activeingredientname=theanine

[198] http://www.ncbi.nlm.nih.gov/pubmed/18296328

[199] The memory-enhancing effects of Euphoria longan fruit extract in mice.

[200] Park, Y. S.; Lee, H. S.; Won, M. H.; Lee, J. H.; Lee, S. Y.; Lee, H. Y. (2002). "Effect of an exo-polysaccharide from the culture broth of Hericium erinaceus on enhancement of growth and differentiation of rat adrenal nerve cells". *Cytotechnology* **39** (3): 155–162. doi:10.1023/A:1023963509393. PMC 3449638. PMID 19003308. edit

Mori, K.; Inatomi, S.; Ouchi, K.; Azumi, Y.; Tuchida, T. (2009). "Improving effects of the mushroom Yamabushitake (*Hericium erinaceus*) on mild cognitive impairment: a double-blind placebo-controlled clinical trial". *Phytotherapy Research* **23** (3): 367–372. doi:10.1002/ptr.2634. PMID 18844328.

Mori, K.; Obara, Y.; Hirota, M.; Azumi, Y.; Kinugasa, S.; Inatomi, S.; Nakahata, N. (2008). "Nerve Growth Factor-Inducing Activity of Hericium erinaceus in 1321N1 Human Astrocytoma Cells". *Biological & Pharmaceutical Bulletin* **31** (9): 1727–1732. doi:10.1248/bpb.31.1727. PMID 18758067.

Bioactive Substances in YAMABUSHITAKE, the Hericium erinaceum, Fungus, and its Medicinal Utilization, Takashi Mizuno, Shizuoka University.

Kolotushkina, E. V.; Moldavan, M. G.; Voronin, K. Y.; Skibo, G. G. (2003). "The influence of Hericium erinaceus extract on myelination process in vitro". *Fiziolohichnyi zhurnal* **49** (1): 38–45. PMID 12675022.

Peripheral Nerve Regeneration Following Crush Injury to Rat Peroneal Nerve by Aqueous Extract of Medicinal Mushroom Hericium erinaceus (Bull.: Fr) Pers. (Aphyllophoromycetideae), Kah-Hui Wong, Institute of Biological Sciences, Faculty of Science, University of Malaya, Kuala Lumpur 50603, Malaysia.

[201] Le Bail, Jean-Christophe; Pouget, Christelle; Fagnere, Catherine; Basly, Jean-Philippe; Chulia, Albert-Jose; Habrioux, Gerard (2001). "Chalcones are potent inhibitors of aromatase and 17β-hydroxysteroid dehydrogenase activities". *Life Sciences* **68** (7): 751–61. doi:10.1016/S0024-3205(00)00974-7. PMID 11205867.

[202] Xu, Q.; Ma, X.; Liang, X. (2007). "Determination of Astragalosides in the Roots of *Astragalus* spp. Using Liquid Chromatography Tandem Atmospheric Pressure Chemical Ionization Mass Spectrometry". *Phytochemical Analysis* **18** (5): 419–427. doi:10.1002/pca.997. PMID 17624885.

Lin, L. Z.; He, X. G.; Lindenmaier, M.; Nolan, G.; Yang, J.; Cleary, M.; Qiu, S. X.; Cordell, G. A. (2000). "Liquid Chromatography-Electrospray Ionization Mass Spectrometry Study of the Flavonoids of the Roots of *Astragalus mongholicus* and *A. membranaceus*". *Journal of Chromatography A* **876** (1–2): 87–95. doi:10.1016/S0021-9673(00)00149-7. PMID 10823504.

[203] Choi, JG; Moon, M; Jeong, HU; Kim, MC; Kim, SY; Oh, MS (2011). "Cistanches Herba enhances learning and memory by inducing nerve growth factor". *Behavioural brain research* **216** (2): 652–8. doi:10.1016/j.bbr.2010.09.008. PMID 20849880.

[204] 4-Hydroxybenzaldehyde from Gastrodia elata B1. is active in the antioxidation and GABAergic neuromodulation of the rat brain. Jeoung-Hee Ha, Dong-Ung Lee, Jae-Tae Lee, Jin-Sook Kim, Chul-Soon Yong, Jung-Ae Kim, Jung-Sang Ha and Keun- Huh, Journal of Ethnopharmacology, Volume 73, Issues 1-2, November 2000, Pages 329-333, doi:10.1016/S0378-8741(00)00313-5

2,4-Bis(4-hydroxybenzyl) phenol from Gastrodia elata. Naoki Noda, Yukio Kobayashi, Kazumoto Miyahara and Saeko Fukahori, doi:10.1016/0031-9422(95)00051-8

Phenolic compounds from Gastrodia rhizome and relaxant effects of related compounds on isolated smooth muscle preparation. Junko Hayashi, Toshikazu Sekine, Shigeyoshi Deguchi, Qing Lin, Syunji Horie, Shizuko Tsuchiya, Shingo Yano, Kazuo Watanabe and Fumio Ikegami, Phytochemistry, Volume 59, Issue 5, March 2002, Pages 513–519, doi:10.1016/S0031-9422(02)00008-0

[205] Singh B. and Rastogi, R. P. 1969. A reinvestigation of the triterpenes of Centella Asiatica. Phytochemistry 8: 917-921.

Singh, B. and Rastogi, R.P. 1968. Chemical examination of Centalla Asiatica Linn - III. Constitution of brahmic acid. Phytochemistry 7: 1385-1393

Murray, edited by Joseph E. Pizzorno, Jr., Michael T. (2012). *Textbook of natural medicine* (4th ed. ed.). Edinburgh: Churchill Livingstone. p. 650. ISBN 9781437723335.

[206] Winston, David; Steven Maimes (April 2007). *Adaptogens: Herbs for Strength, Stamina, and Stress Relief.* Healing Arts Press. ISBN 978-1-59477-158-3. Contains a detailed herbal monograph on jiaogulan and highlights health benefits.

Bensky, Dan; Andrew Gamble; Steven Clavey; Erich Stöger (September 2004). *Chinese Herbal Medicine: Materia Medica, 3rd Edition.* Eastland Press. ISBN 978-0-939616-42-8.

[208] http://www.fasebj.org/cgi/content/meeting_abstract/26/1_MeetingAbstracts/112.8

[209] Lee J.-Y., Kim K.Y., Shin K.Y., Won B.Y., Jung H.Y., Suh Y.H. (2009). "Effects of BT-11 on memory in healthy humans". *Neuroscience Letters* **454** (2): 111–114. doi:10.1016/j.neulet.2009.03.024. PMID 19429065.

[210] Shin K.Y., Lee J.-Y., Won B.Y., Jung H.Y., Chang K.-A., Koppula S., Suh Y.-H. (2009). "BT-11 is effective for enhancing cognitive functions in the elderly humans". *Neuroscience Letters* **465** (2): 157–159. doi:10.1016/j.neulet.2009.08.033.

[211] Yabe T., Tuchida H., Kiyohara H., Takeda T., Yamada H. (2003). "Induction of NGF synthesis in astrocytes by onjisaponins of *Polygala tenuifolia*, constituents of kampo (Japanese herbal) medicine, Ninjin-yoei-to.". *Phytomedicine* **10** (2-3): 106–14. doi:10.1078/094471103321659799. PMID 12725562.

[212] Jin Zeng-liang L., Gao Nana, Zhang Jian-rui R., et al (2014). "The discovery of Yuanzhi-1, a triterpenoid saponin derived from the traditional Chinese medicine, has antidepressant-like activity". *Progress in neuro-psychopharmacology & biological psychiatry.* **53**: 9–14. doi:10.1016/j.pnpbp.2014.02.013.

[213] Hu Yuan, Liu Ming, Liu Ping, Guo Dai-Hong H., Wei Ri-Bao B., Rahman Khalid. (2011). "Possible mechanism of the antidepressant effect of 3,6'-disinapoyl sucrose from Polygala tenuifolia Willd". *The Journal of pharmacy and pharmacology* **63**: 869–874. doi:10.1111/j.2042-7158.2011.01281.x.

[214] Xue Wei, Hu Jin-feng, Yuan Yu-he, et al. (2009). "Polygalasaponin XXXII from Polygala tenuifolia root improves hippocampal-dependent learning and memory". *Acta Pharmacologica* **30**: 1211–1219. doi:10.1038/aps.2009.112.

[215] Hu Yuan, Liao Hong-Bo, Liu Ping, Dai-Hong Guo, Wang Yu-Yu, Rahman Khalid. (2009). "Antidepressant-like effects of 3,6'-disinapoyl sucrose on hippocampal neuronal plasticity and neurotrophic signal pathway in chronically mild stressed rats". *Neurochemistry International.* doi:10.1016/j.neuint.2009.12.004

[216] Cheong Myung-Hee H., Lee Sang-Ryong R., Yoo Hwa-Seung S., et al. (2011). "Anti-inflammatory effects of Polygala tenuifolia root through inhibition of NF-κB activation in lipopolysaccharide-induced BV2 microglial cells.". *Journal of Ethnopharmacology.* doi:10.1016/j.jep.2011.08.008.

[217] http://www.itmonline.org/arts/rehmann.htm

[218] Liu, J; He QJ; Zou W; Wang HX; Bao YM; Liu YX; An LJ (December 2006). "Catalpol increases hippocampal neuroplasticity and up-regulates PKC and BDNF in the aged rats". *Brain Research* **1123** (1): 68–79. doi:10.1016/j.brainres.2006.09.058. PMID 17078935.

[219] http://www.itmonline.org/kunzle/rosemary.htm

[221] http://www.medicalnewstoday.com/releases/87172.php

[222] Altun A, Ugur-Altun B (May 2007). "Melatonin: therapeutic and clinical utilization". *Int. J. Clin. Pract.* **61** (5): 835–45. doi:10.1111/j.1742-1241.2006.01191.x. PMID 17298593.

[223] Hardeland R (July 2005). "Antioxidative protection by melatonin: multiplicity of mechanisms from radical detoxification to radical avoidance". *Endocrine* **27** (2): 119–30. doi:10.1385/ENDO:27:2:119. PMID 16217125.

[224] Marx CE, Bradford DW, Hamer RM, et al. (September 2011). "Pregnenolone as a novel therapeutic candidate in schizophrenia: emerging preclinical and clinical evidence". *Neuroscience* **191**: 78–90. doi:10.1016/j.neuroscience.2011.06.076. PMID 21756978

[225] Teufel A, Malik N, Mukhopadhyay M, Westphal H (2002). "Frcp1 and Frcp2, two novel fibronectin type III repeat containing genes". *Gene* **297** (1–2): 79–83. doi:10.1016/S0378-1119(02)00828-4. PMID 12384288.

Ferrer-Martínez A, Ruiz-Lozano P, Chien KR (2002). "Mouse PeP: A novel peroxisomal protein linked to myoblast differentiation and development". *Developmental Dynamics* **224** (2): 154–167. doi:10.1002/dvdy.10099. PMID 12112469

[226] Erickson HP (2013). "Irisin and FNDC5 in retrospect: An exercise hormone or a transmembrane receptor?". *Adipocyte* **2** (4): 289–293. doi:10.4161/adip.26082. PMC 3774709. PMID 24052909

[227] http://www.nia.nih.gov/research/dab/interventions-testing-program-itp/compounds-testing

[228] Bian, M. T. [Determination of 10-hydroxy-2-decenoic acid in ginseng royal jelly by reversed phase high performance liquid chromatography]. Chung Yao Tung Pao. 12(6):41-43, 1987.

Bloodworth, BC; Harn, CS; Hock, CT; Boon, YO (Jul–Aug 1995). "Liquid chromatographic determination of trans-10-hydroxy-2-decenoic acid content of commercial products containing royal jelly.". *Journal of AOAC International* **78** (4): 1019–23. PMID 7580313.

Genç, Mahmut; Aslan, Abdurrahman. "Determination of trans-10-hydroxy-2-decenoic acid content in pure royal jelly and royal jelly products by column liquid chromatography". *Journal of Chromatography A* **839** (1-2): 265–268. doi:10.1016/S0021-9673(99)00151-X. PMID 10327631.

Ji, N; Yu, RG; Yang, QH; Yu, PH; Li, Y (Jul 1987). "[Determination of 10-hydroxy-trans-2-decenoic acid (10-HDA) in royal jelly by gas liquid chromatography].". *Zhong yao tong bao (Beijing, China : 1981)* **12** (9): 28–31, 62. PMID 3449246.

[229] Royal Jelly and Its Unique Fatty Acid, 10-Hydroxy-Trans-2-Decenoic Acid, Promote Neurogenesis by Neural Stem/progenitor Cells in Vitro. Biomedical Research (Tokyo, Japan) 28(5): 261–266.

[230] 10-Hydroxy-2-decenoic acid, a unique medium-chain fatty acid, activates 5'-AMP-activated protein kinase in L6 myotubes and mice. Mol Nutr Food Res. 2013 Oct;57(10):1794–802.

[231] http://jonlieffmd.com/blog/polyunsaturated-fatty-acid-signaling-in-the-brain

[232] Brain Cephalin, a mixture of Phosphatides. Separation from it of Phosphatidyl serine, Phosphatidyl ethanolamine, and a fraction containing an inositol Phosphatide

[233] *Neuron.* 2010 Jan 28;65(2):165-77.

[234] http://www.nature.com/news/testing-magnesium-s-brain-boosting-effects-1.11665

http://www.magtein.com/

[235] Sartori HE (1986). "Lithium orotate in the treatment of alcoholism and related conditions". *Alcohol.* **3** (2): 97–100. doi:10.1016/0741-8329(86)90018-2. PMID 3718672.

Schrauzer GN, Shrestha KP (May 1990). "Lithium in drinking water and the incidences of crimes, suicides, and arrests related to drug addictions". *Biol Trace Elem Res.* **25** (2): 105–13. doi:10.1007/bf02990271. PMID 1699579.

Helbich M, Leitner M, Kapusta ND (Jun 2012). "Geospatial examination of lithium in drinking water and suicide mortality". *Int J Health Geogr.* **11**: 19. doi:10.1186/1476-072X-11-19. PMID 22695110

[236] Flynn, B. L.; Ranno, A. E. (February 1999). "Pharmacologic Management of Alzheimer Disease, Part II: Antioxidants, Antihypertensives, and Ergoloid Derivatives". *Annals of Pharmacotherapy* **33** (2): 188–197. doi:10.1345/aph.17172. PMID 10084415.

[237] Schneider, L. S.; Olin, J. T. (August 1994). "Overview of Clinical Trials of Hydergine in Dementia". *Archives of Neurology* **51** (8): 787–798. doi:10.1001/archneur.1994.00540200063018. PMID 8042927.

[238] Suno M, Nagaoka A. Inhibition of lipid peroxidation by a novel compound (CV-2619) in brain mitochondria and mode of action of the inhibition. *Biochem Biophys Res Commun.* (1984)

[239]

http://www.webmd.com/vitamins-supplements/ingredientmono-1078-idebenone.aspx?activeingredientid=1078&activeingredientname=idebenone

http://www.ncbi.nlm.nih.gov/pubmed/9215809

[240] http://www.ncbi.nlm.nih.gov/pubmed/7824194

http://www.ncbi.nlm.nih.gov/pubmed/1347497

[241] Alvarez-Guerra M, Bertholom N, Garay RP (1999). "Selective blockade by nicergoline of vascular responses elicited by stimulation of alpha 1A-adrenoceptor subtype in the rat". *Fundam Clin Pharmacol* **13** (1): 50–8. doi:10.1111/j.1472-8206.1999.tb00320.x. PMID 10027088.

[242] PatentGenius.com http://www.patentgenius.com/patent/5439930.html

[243] ROZANTSEV GRIGORI G, SKOLDINOV ALEXANDER P, TROPHIMOV SERGEI S, HALIKAS JAMES A, GARIBOVA TAISIJA L. Biologically active n-acylprolydipeptides having antiamnestic, antihypoxic and anorexigenic effects. US5439930 (A) 1995-08-08.

[244] Institute of Molecular Genetics, Russian Academy of Sciences website (http://old.img.ras.ru/semax1-e.htm)

[245] http://www.ncbi.nlm.nih.gov/pubmed/11569188

[246] http://www.scirp.org/journal/PaperInformation.aspx?PaperID=40560#.U9VYWfldVWg

http://www.sciencedirect.com/science/article/pii/S0006899306022955

http://link.springer.com/article/10.1023%2FA%3A1025177812262

[247] Sakamoto T, Cansev M, Wurtman RJ. Oral supplementation with docosahexaenoic acid and uridine-5′-monophosphate increases dendritic spine density in adult gerbil hippocampus. Brain Res. 2007 Nov 28;1182:50-9.

Drees F, Gertler FB. Ena/VASP: proteins at the tip of the nervous system. Curr Opin Neurobiol. 2008 Feb;18(1):53-9.

Yamauchi T. Molecular mechanism of learning and memory based on the research for Ca2+/calmodulin-dependent protein kinase II. Yakugaku Zasshi. 2007 Aug;127(8):1173-97.

Skaper SD. Neuronal growth-promoting and inhibitory cues in neuroprotection and neuroregeneration. Ann NY Acad Sci. 2005 Aug;1053:376-85.

[248] http://www.ncbi.nlm.nih.gov/pubmed/21379380

http://www.ncbi.nlm.nih.gov/pubmed/8687475

[249] Ashour OM, Naguib FN, el Kouni MH. 5-(m-Benzyloxybenzyl)barbituric acid acyclonucleoside, a uridine phosphorylase inhibitor, and 2',3',5'-tri-O-acetyluridine, a prodrug of uridine, as modulators of plasma uridine concentration. Implications for chemotherapy. *Biochem Pharmacol.* (1996)

[250] http://www.ncbi.nlm.nih.gov/pubmed/11722606

http://www.ncbi.nlm.nih.gov/pubmed/11418861

http://www.ncbi.nlm.nih.gov/pubmed/16365320

http://www.ncbi.nlm.nih.gov/pubmed/22528682

http://www.ncbi.nlm.nih.gov/pubmed/14699960

[251] Arabbi PR, Genovese MI, Lajolo FM. Flavonoids in vegetable foods commonly consumed in Brazil and estimated ingestion by the Brazilian population. *J Agric Food Chem.* (2004)

Careri M, *et al.* Direct HPLC analysis of quercetin and trans-resveratrol in red wine, grape, and winemaking byproducts. *J Agric Food Chem.* (2003)

[252] Liu X, Chan CB, Jang SW, Pradoldej S, Huang J, He K et al. (2010). "A synthetic 7,8-dihydroxyflavone derivative promotes neurogenesis and exhibits potent antidepressant effect". *J. Med. Chem.* **53** (23): 8274–86. doi:10.1021/jm101206p. PMC 3150605. PMID 21073191

[253] Castello NA, Nguyen MH, Tran JD, Cheng D, Green KN, LaFerla FM (2014). "7,8-Dihydroxyflavone, a small molecule TrkB agonist, improves spatial memory and increases thin spine density in a mouse model of Alzheimer disease-like neuronal loss". *PLoS ONE* **9** (3): e91453. doi:10.1371/journal.pone.0091453. PMC 3948846. PMID 24614170.

Chen C, Li XH, Zhang S, Tu Y, Wang YM, Sun HT (2014). "7,8-dihydroxyflavone ameliorates scopolamine-induced Alzheimer-like pathologic dysfunction". *Rejuvenation Res* **17** (3): 249–54. doi:10.1089/rej.2013.1519. PMID 24325271.

Zhang Z, Liu X, Schroeder JP, Chan CB, Song M, Yu SP et al. (2014). "7,8-dihydroxyflavone prevents synaptic loss and memory deficits in a mouse model of Alzheimer's disease". *Neuropsychopharmacology* **39** (3): 638–50. doi:10.1038/npp.2013.243. PMID 24022672.

[254] Yang YJ, Li YK, Wang W, Wan JG, Yu B, Wang MZ et al. (2014). "Small-molecule TrkB agonist 7,8-dihydroxyflavone reverses cognitive and synaptic plasticity deficits in a rat model of schizophrenia". *Pharmacol. Biochem. Behav.* **122**: 30–6. doi:10.1016/j.pbb.2014.03.013. PMID 24662915.

[255] Jang SW, Liu X, Yepes M, Shepherd KR, Miller GW, Liu Y et al. (2010). "A selective TrkB agonist with potent neurotrophic activities by 7,8-dihydroxyflavone". *Proc. Natl. Acad. Sci. U.S.A.* **107** (6): 2687–92. doi:10.1073/pnas.0913572107. PMC 2823863. PMID 20133810.

[256] Jiang M, Peng Q, Liu X, Jin J, Hou Z, Zhang J et al. (2013). "Small-molecule TrkB receptor agonists improve motor function and extend survival in a mouse model of Huntington's disease". *Hum. Mol. Genet.* **22** (12): 2462–70. doi:10.1093/hmg/ddt098. PMC 3658168. PMID 23446639.

257 Korkmaz OT, Aytan N, Carreras I, Choi JK, Kowall NW, Jenkins BG et al. (2014). "7,8-Dihydroxyflavone improves motor performance and enhances lower motor neuronal survival in a mouse model of amyotrophic lateral sclerosis". *Neurosci. Lett.* **566**: 286–91. doi:10.1016/j.neulet.2014.02.058. PMID 24637017

258 Wu CH, Hung TH, Chen CC, Ke CH, Lee CY, Wang PY et al. (2014). "Post-injury treatment with 7,8-dihydroxyflavone, a TrkB receptor agonist, protects against experimental traumatic brain injury via PI3K/Akt signaling". *PLoS ONE* **9** (11): e113397. doi:10.1371/journal.pone.0113397. PMC 4240709. PMID 25415296.

259 Wang B, Wu N, Liang F, Zhang S, Ni W, Cao Y et al. (2014). "7,8-dihydroxyflavone, a small-molecule tropomyosin-related kinase B (TrkB) agonist, attenuates cerebral ischemia and reperfusion injury in rats". *J. Mol. Histol.* **45** (2): 129–40. doi:10.1007/s10735-013-9539-y. PMID 24045895.

Uluc K, Kendigelen P, Fidan E, Zhang L, Chanana V, Kintner D et al. (2013). "TrkB receptor agonist 7, 8 dihydroxyflavone triggers profound gender- dependent neuroprotection in mice after perinatal hypoxia and ischemia". *CNS Neurol Disord Drug Targets* **12** (3): 360–70. PMC 3674109. PMID 23469848.

260 Sánchez L, Calvo M, Brock JH (1992). "Biological role of lactoferrin". *Arch. Dis. Child.* **67** (5): 657–61. doi:10.1136/adc.67.5.657. PMC 1793702. PMID 1599309.

261 Tayyem RF, Heath DD, Al-Delaimy WK, Rock CL (2006). "Curcumin content of turmeric and curry powders". *Nutr Cancer* **55** (2): 126–131. doi:10.1207/s15327914nc5502_2. PMID 17044766.

262 Mosley, Michael. "Unexpected ways to wake up your brain". *bbc.co.uk*. BBC. Retrieved 30 October 2014.